Coping Skills Manual for Treating Chronic and Terminal Illness

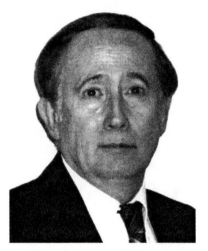

Kenneth Sharoff, PhD, has been practicing psychotherapy for 30 years, and is currently in private practice in Phoenix, Maryland. He received his BA from the University of Colorado, his MA from the University of Denver, and his PhD from the University of Maryland. He is the originator of cognitive coping therapy, reviewed as "the most important contribution in the development and maturing of cognitive behavior therapy in the past 20 years." He lives with his wife, two children, and assorted pets.

Coping Skills Manual
for Treating Chronic
and Terminal Illness

Kenneth Sharoff, PhD

 Springer Publishing Company

Springer Publishing Company, Inc.
536 Broadway
New York, NY 10012-3955

Acquisitions Editor: Sheri W. Sussman
Production Editor: Jeanne W. Libby
Cover design by: Joanne Honigman

01 02 03 04 05/5 4 3 2 1

Library of Congress Cataloging-in-Publication Data

Sharoff, Kenneth.
Coping skills manual for treating chronic and terminal illness / by Kenneth Sharoff.
    p. cm.
   Includes bibliographical references.
   ISBN 0-8261-2276-0
   Chronic diseases—Psychological aspects. 2. Terminal care. 3. Cognitive therapy. 4. Adjustment (Psychology)
   5. Terminally ill—Mental health. I. Title.
RC108.S47 2004
362.196'044—dc22   2004002649

Printed in the United States of America by Integrated Book Technology.

This book is dedicated to my wife, Nancy,
who has demonstrated to me how to live with chronic pain
with dignity and grace.

Contents

Introduction

With the development of a chronic or terminal illness, many people suddenly find themselves unable to use the skills that they had previously learned for managing life problems and securing what they want. Their skill repertoire is incomplete, insufficient, or it contains skills and strategies that are inappropriate for adapting to a chronic or terminal illness.

However, once medical patients learn skills necessary to adjust to their condition, the illness may not seem so intimidating, overwhelming, onerous, and taxing. Disease, at that point, becomes another factor—although a major factor—in the life of the person.

This book helps providers address treatment issues that arise when developing the skills necessary for living with disease and treatment. It focuses on health provider concerns in their work with patients. An accompanying text, *Coping Skills Therapy for Managing Chronic and Terminal Illness* (Sharoff, 2004, Springer Publishing) discusses the specific skills themselves in much greater detail and presents a guide to treat various treatment issues regarding a coping skills approach. Sharoff (2002) has previously expanded the use of coping skills therapy for psychotherapy and has termed his approach Cognitive Coping Therapy (CCT). This manual extends his work into the health care area.

Supplying people with coping skills helps to develop healthy functioning. Instinctively people work to employ a way to cope to eliminate the problems that they encounter (Wine, 1980; Snyder & Dinoff, 1999), however our concern is whether their way of coping is adaptive, rational, and realistic. While people cope in their own way, that way may not be the best for themselves or others. Pathology is therefore viewed as a coping strategy that is not producing the best results. Pathology may result when people habitually fail to get where they want to go, because they select the wrong way to get there.

Providers need to assess that issue. Do patients have the means to get where they want to go, or have they selected the wrong way to get there? As a tool, a skill can be adapted for any situation. There is no such thing as a "bad" or harmful coping skill. There are only bad or harmful coping strategies. When patients with a psychological disorder come to therapy, a skill may appear dysfunctional but that can be because of how it is used. Utilized in a different way or different context and supplemented with other skills, that same ability can be very beneficial.

INTENT OF BOOK

This book is a practical guide for implementing a coping skills approach and discusses the theory and techniques of cognitive coping therapy with chronic and terminally ill patients. It also lists techniques for a variety of problems and illustrates how a coping skills program can help with that problem. The manual and CD are meant to stand alone as a guide for practitioners.

At the same time the manual does not fully elucidate and explain those skills. That is beyond the scope of this book, which is meant to be a companion to *Coping Skills Therapy for Managing Chronic and Terminal Illness* (henceforth referred to as the Coping Skills Book in this text). Therein the reader will find more detailed descriptions of the skills and tactics of CCT.

The Manual seeks to guide practitioners in using a coping skills approach. It illuminates treatment issues and problems that can arise when implementing a skill, such as patient resistance (see chapters 6 and 10). The Manual presents several assessment tools in chapters 5, 6, and 10. It discusses how to diagnose a patient from a skills perspective (chapter 2). Ways to treat maladaptive coping strategies (chapter 3) are discussed. Throughout the Manual other modalities are utilized, such as Gestalt, solutions-oriented therapy, and paradoxical therapy, to show readers how to intermix techniques and orientations from other perspectives. A coping skills approach is part of cognitive-behavioral therapy (CBT), which also includes cognitive restructuring (CR). Chapter 4 discusses this approach in detail to familiarize readers with this method. The Manual lists the benefits and limitations of CR with medical patients.

The Manual also provides therapists with assessment instruments and handouts that can be given to patients and are available on the accompanying compact disc. The notation *** will be seen in the Manual to indicate that part of the text is on the disc.

PROSPECTIVE THERAPY

Coping skills therapy is a *prospective form of treatment.* It looks forward in time and plots the steps needed to accomplish a goal. One skill needs other skills to be successful. This model of care approaches people like they were a construction project, where one part of a project needs to be put in place before another part can be erected, to create a sound, well-built structure. Each "human structure" is a highly individualized project, where the skills necessary to attain a goal are developed based on the unique characteristics and personality of that person.

The beginning of treatment starts with a series of questions: The first questions concern the issue of goals: What do you want for yourself? Where do you want to be heading? To help patients reach their goals, the focus then shifts to the skills needed to attain those goals (e.g., "I hear this disease has caused you to be deprived in many ways, but do you have ability to tolerate deprivation when it occurs?").

The next group of questions concerns the issue of external or internal barriers keeping people from reaching their goals, and where people are stuck in the process of goal attainment. Process questions are posed, such as: If you are stuck, where are you stuck? What's keeping you stuck? How is that barrier keeping you from getting what you want? What is keeping you from moving aside those barriers? Process questions illuminate the cycle perpetuating the problem. The intention is to change the cycle by implanting a capacity, removing an inappropriate response, or performing a response at an appropriate level for the purpose of overcoming the barrier or stuck point.

The ability to chain responses requires a predictive ability and "what if" curiosity. Therapists need to continuously asks themselves, "If X is initiated, what will happen next and what will need to be in place to manage that situation?" Coping skills therapists must be *proactive* and install needed responses before it becomes obvious that a given response is needed.

To operate as a coping skills therapist, *providers will assume several roles.* They will be an educator as they teach a skill, and a trainer and coach to develop skill proficiency. They will act as a director, selecting and encouraging the use of that response in various situations. A coping skills therapist must be comfortable being an active therapist.

If patients shun or ignore implementing a skill, then this illustrates that another coping strategy (that may or may not be effective or adaptive) is in effect and other skills (that may or may not be appropriate) are being used for managing in a given situation. In that case providers need to identify the prevailing strategy and the skills being used.

In CCT, therapists are strongly advised to view resistance as a coping strategy. The benefits and drawbacks of that strategy are identified and then patients are asked to choose if they want to continue using that strategy. This forces responsibility-taking onto patients for whatever problems arise from using a strategy and set of skills in a particular way. Alternative strategies to the resistance are then given along with their benefits and drawbacks. When presenting new strategies and skills therapists need to be adept at marketing. They need to know how to induct and motivate patients into using that ability.

COGNITIVE FORMATION OF SKILLS

Skills are formed out of a cognitive process (Sharoff, 2002, 2004). First a skill is employed because of a *policy belief* about a situation. The policy sets the position on an issue, a rule for a situation, or a plan about how to do something. Once the policy is formed, self-instructions are formed to carry it out. The self-instructions give specific rules, guidelines, permissions, and prohibitions about how to act regarding a policy. CCT refers to them as an **executive belief**, because they are thoughts about how to execute the policy or a given coping response. They direct a person in how to think, what to perceive, how to manage emotion, and how to act. They mostly operate on a subconscious level. The content of thinking is referred to as an **operational belief**. They are formed by the executive beliefs that the influence the content of thinking. People are aware of their operational beliefs.

CCT maintains that the heart of pathology comes from the executive beliefs, when they are ill-formed, inappropriate, or maladaptive. CCT puts more emphasis on them than the policy beliefs, which is the primary concern of cognitive restructurists.

TREATMENT TACTICS

A coping skills model can employ one of several tactics.

1) RESPONSE SUBSTITUTION TACTIC

This is the most common tactic used in CCT. A determination is made that a response is problematic and another response is formulated that can lead to the desired outcome (Bandura, 1969). That response is then substituted for the maladaptive or incorrect response. A maladaptive response does not lead to adjustment of the problem. Oppositely, an adaptive response does not change the situation but allows a person to tolerate and accommodate to it so there is less negative emotion. An incorrect response does not fit the context.

An example of a response substitution tactic is when there is rejection of further suffering and the patient learns to assimilate suffering. In place of the former the latter is installed, which allows patients to co-exist with their distress instead of hating to be that way. Assertiveness training is a response substitution for passive or aggressive expression. Other examples include acting like a role model or acting out a desired outcome in place of a problematic behavior.

2) RESPONSE FACILITATION TACTIC

A response is initiated to encourage a series of other desired responses. An example is symbolic gesturing (Sharoff, 2004), where a physical gesture is implemented (e.g., both hands are raised slowly and open-up to the surroundings) to bring about a different attitude (e.g., to be receptive to undesirable events without feeling resentful). Imagery is used quite often to spark a desired response (Sheikh, 1983).

3) RESPONSE PREVENTION TACTIC

In this tactic, a response is not allowed, is inhibited, or delayed and that allows another response to emerge in its place. For example, *self-instruction training* is used to keep someone from doing something (e.g., "Don't get tense in this situation."). *Symbolic gesturing* can be used for this purpose (e.g., the hands move down to stand for termination of angry rumination.).

4) STIMULUS SUBSTITUTION TACTIC

One stimulus (or series of stimuli) replaces another stimulus that is problematic. For example, **sensory diversion training** (Sharoff, 2002, 2004) is utilized to substitute for a troublesome stimulus. One sense is selected and it focuses on a series of neutral or positive stimuli instead of dealing with one that results in distress. **Psychological distancing** is another example of a stimulus substitution (Sharoff, 2004). In this skill one stimulus substitutes for another. For example, instead of responding to the stimulus directly a person sees him/herself from a different vantagepoint, such as looking at oneself on stage from the audience when anxious or angry. This simultaneously changes the stimulus. Also, psychological distancing is another way to gain objectivity and calmness, because it switches activity from the limbic region of the brain to the cerebral cortex.

5) STIMULUS PREVENTION TACTIC

A stimulus is not allowed to occur or its activity is controlled in some way. An example is **thought stopping**, which halts a thought by strongly saying "Stop" when distress builds (Wolpe, 1969). Another example is the Zen technique of "**No mind—no thing**," which operates to obliterate all thoughts on the mind (Watts, 1965). In each case, without influencing the stimulus, a different response can occur.

SUMMARY

A coping skills approach gives people tools to get what they want. Psychopathology does the same thing, and therapists need to identify the skills in the pathological response to benefit the patient. A skills approach is a prospective form of treatment, constructing response chains to attain a goal. The executive beliefs provide instructions on how to execute the skill. There are tactics that are employed to utilize skills; most common is the response substitution tactic.

Theory of Pathology and Health

In this chapter, providers will learn how to diagnose their patients from a coping skills perspective. The chapter also presents skills that are instrumental for leading to healthy functioning.

THEORY OF PATHOLOGY

Cognitive Coping Therapy (CCT) views psychopathology and dysfunction from a coping skills standpoint. It maintains that pathology is due to either a skills deficit or an error in usage.

COPING SKILLS DEFICIT

Disease is exacerbating enough, but if key skills are lacking or are insufficient then the hardship becomes much more severe. Goals cannot be attained, causing the troublesome situations to be viewed more harshly. Oppositely, when goals are attained disease feels less onerous and overwhelming.

A lack of skill is referred to as a coping skill deficit. It may appear in several ways. One, a lack of skills existed prior to the onset of illness. Pre-morbid adjustment was already poor in some way, which in turn results in a poor adjustment when new challenges like disease arise. Two, a patient may have good coping ability in general but has deficient ability in certain areas, which becomes a problem when there is ill health. Three, a patient may have some components of an ability but lack one or more of its component skills, and that results in dysfunction.

COPING SKILLS EXCESS

Many times an individual has a legitimate, helpful, useful skill but uses it excessively in a particular situation or across situations. In essence, the maxim is practiced: if something works do more of it and that will yield even better results. If a solution is not producing the desired results then use more and more of that solution in the hope of resolving the problem. But, the excessive use of a solution can become a problem in and of itself (Watzlawick, Weakland, & Fisch, 1974), and CCT refers to this as a coping skills excess.

Decreasing a coping skills excess can be very difficult for many patients. Because the more-of-the-same solution has worked in the past that reinforces its continued use in the future. In addition, the coping skills excess strategy often becomes a personality trait and part of someone's identity. It feels comfortable being that way while being different seems like acting "out-of-character." In general, people stick to what they know, even if it hurts them.

CONTEXTUALIZATION ERROR

People can commit two types of contextualization errors. One is where the meaning for a situation does not fit that context. The facts refute the meaning but the person continues to believe that the meaning is correct. A second contextualization error is where a skill is used in the wrong context. The skill is appropriate, beneficial, and used in an appropriate amount (so it would not be a coping skills excess), but it should not be employed in a particular setting.

Many cardiac patients commit a contextualization error in both meaning and coping strategy for their situation. After a heart attack there are often many painful changes in bodily condition that comprise stable or classical angina. Yet, this condition is not usually dangerous. A problem arises when cardiac patients mistake their routine angina symptoms for another heart attack, rush to the emergency room, and see their cardiologist unnecessarily. The problem: the meaning does not match the context, the situation the person is in.

The contextualization problem continues when angina patients feel frightened about having another heart attack, so they adopt a coping response that in their mind minimizes any chance of that occurring. They become inactive, which causes them to become deconditioned, which in turn strains their heart even more. They scrutinize their body for any sign of trouble. They become hypervigilant. The consequence is an increase in anxiety that strains their heart even more. To avoid any strain on their heart, they often stop working and stop participating in hobbies that previously gave them meaning, causing them to lose satisfaction with their life. Many cardiologists refer to this group of angina patients pejoratively as "cardiac cripples." Their highly cautious, overly careful coping response is inappropriate for stable angina but appropriate for unstable angina, which is more of an acute, dangerous condition, or any precarious, unstable medical problem.

TIME-FIT ERRORS

People develop many skills from earlier periods in their life, in particular from childhood. Those skills are then carried into the present or adulthood mindlessly. They are taken for granted and performed mechanically because they have been around for so long. In those earlier contexts those skills did help the person cope and manage. Problems arise when early life coping skills are not consciously evaluated for applicability and suitability in the present. When previous life skills not appropriate for the present context continue to be used, CCT refers to this as a time-fit error. While once helpful they are no longer efficacious.

Once earlier life skills become entrenched there is great difficulty surrendering their use. People feel loyal to strategies that got them through hard times in the past, even though that same strategy is counterproductive in the present. Yet, an early life skill does not have to be abandoned entirely, because it may have utility elsewhere. Providers need to assess what skills are required for the patient's present situation and seek redeployment of previously learned skills for other settings. Many early life skills appear dysfunctional but if they can be refined, refitted, or combined with other skills then they can have merit.

SEQUENCING ERROR

Coping skills are comprised of several subskills. Those subskills need to be performed in the right sequence or else additional problems can occur. CCT refers to skills being used in the wrong order as a sequencing error.

Many patients entering long-term care facilities often commit sequencing errors. Forced to leave their homes and enter the facility because of an unstable medical condition, they feel frightened. To cope they first withdraw and become detached but do not investigate if there are reasons for being frightened. They presume danger of one sort or another is present before getting to know if that conclusion is warranted. While not finding any signs of danger many continue to avoid making contact with others. As a consequence, their adaptation to the long-term care facility goes poorly. The problem: useful coping strategy (avoidance) but used in the wrong sequence.

What would be the appropriate sequence? First assess the situation for danger. If none is found then venture forth and experience the situation. Become involved in it and see if it is dangerous or unsatisfying. If that turns out to be the case then withdraw and avoid contact, but do not take that step prematurely.

IRRATIONAL, MALADAPTIVE COPING SKILL

There are many skills that when used individually cause no problem. Problems arise though, when those same skills are coupled with other skills and the interaction of them interferes with adaptation.

CCT refers to those unproductive combinations of skills as an irrational, maladaptive coping skill (IMCS). Yet, people continue to use an IMCS because it does provide some measure of coping. Chapter 10 discusses the components of an IMCS.

THEORY OF HEALTH

Sharoff (2002) has previously identified a set of skills that lead to maximum adjustment and healthy functioning. Those skills are acceptance, tolerance, mourning, self-support, descriptive judgments, problem solving, perceptual shifting, and self-assurance. In addition, the skill of accommodation is recommended for medical patients when appropriate. Following is a brief introduction to each of these skills.

Acceptance

This ability consists of recognition of reality, allowing reality into one's life on intellectual and emotional levels, and co-existing with reality without protesting, rejecting, or passionately hating it. This means coming to terms with boundaries—one's own, those of another person, and those imposed by the disease.

Tolerance

This is an ability to withstand or bear something beyond one's control. It is practiced even if someone works to change a troublesome situation (thus taking a nonsurrender strategy), because the disagreeable situation still has to be endured until it is changed.

Mourning

This is an ability to grieve for losses inherent in a situation. There are several mourning tasks. One task is experiencing the sadness, which is an ability to face and feel psychological pain for a period of time. A second task is summoning various parts of self to engage in the mourning process, such as the emotions, the intellect, or an inspiring capacity to push on while in pain. To be adept in this, the skill of **constructive mourning** is proposed (Sharoff, 2002, 2004).

Self-Support

This is an ability to boost self-esteem, build optimism, concentrate attention on positive qualities, be an advocate for oneself, and relate to oneself in a caring, loving manner.

Descriptive Judging

This is an ability to learn about the situation on its own merits by using a phenomenological investigation (Zinker, 1977). Evaluative restraint is first practiced to halt the urge to rate before describing. Empirically based evidence then is collected about the situation to guide actions, as a prelude to confirming or disconfirming incorrect beliefs about a situation.

Problem Solving

This is an ability to first define the problem and then select alternative solutions to resolve it. The consequences from those solutions are then identified. One solution is selected followed by identifying the tactics to operationalize that solution (D'Zurilla & Goldfried, 1971; Goldfried, 1980; Mahoney & Arnkoff, 1978; Spivack, Platt, & Shure, 1976).

Perceptual Shifting

This is an ability to shift perception on to other matters instead of staying fixed on a negative foreground image presently dominating attention. Other parts of the whole experience are noted besides the negative matter at hand.

Self-Assurance

This is an ability to formulate positive self-images, where the self is viewed as capable and able to accomplish goals. Self-assurance is not just a feeling about oneself but a mental ability to set self-perception and the view of the outcome—before it actually occurs. It creates what Bandura (1977, 1997) calls self-efficacy, the belief that the individual can affect the consequences of a situation.

Accommodation

This is an ability to adjust to a problematic situation or a negative feeling that keeps recurring. At the same time undesirable forces exist a philosophy is established to co-exist with them.

SUMMARY

CCT proposes a theory of pathology based on coping skills deficits and errors in using skills. Coping skill errors include a coping skills excess, a contextualization error, a time-fit error, and a sequencing error. An improper combination of skills is referred to as an irrational maladaptive coping skill. A theory of health for medical patients is proposed that includes the following skills: acceptance, tolerance, mourning, self-support, descriptive judging, problem solving, perceptual shifting, self-assurance, and accommodation.

Chapter 3

Strategies for Disease

Cognitive Coping Therapy (CCT) explicitly assumes that human beings must plan their lives. Entering a situation, they immediately form a strategy about how to fulfill a need, secure a goal, or execute an objective. The strategy sets the over all plan and conduct for functioning in a given situation.

Once the strategy has been selected, the next step is to deploy skills required to accomplish it. Skills are the means to reach the end-goal. To do this, people utilize a metacognitive ability that is termed a *master skill*. It identifies and configures which skills will be necessary and helpful. It arranges the sequence for using them so they form a coordinated maneuver to gain the end-goal. In summary, skills are part of the tactics utilized to secure the objective designated by the strategic plan.

Strategies need to be evaluated by the results that they bring about: does the strategy aid or hinder adaptation? The goal of a strategy is greatly influenced by when it is used. For instance, in the initial stage of disease a strategy can produce harm but in the later phase of disease that same strategy can aid adaptation.

This chapter focuses on common maladaptive strategies, and how and when they have applicability. The chapter also includes what skills need to be added to a maladaptive strategy to avoid a harmful outcome. CCT encourages therapists not to view a strategy with prejudice or alarm but rather to see it as something that has potential for benefit, depending on when it is used, and how it is modified and utilized.

DENIAL STRATEGY

Someone who pursues a strategy of denial copes by having no crisis. Symptoms arise—vision blurs, limbs tingle, the skin turns yellow, lumps are felt—but the denier remains in a psychological cocoon, running his or her life as if nothing has happened differently.

How is this possible when the body is experiencing obvious problems? One way denial can occur is by refusing to recognize what is being felt or observed. Facts are ignored, overlooked, or rejected. The denier goes on as if nothing is wrong: see no evil, hear no evil. Second, denial can occur when a symptom arises but it is not given any particular meaning. It then becomes another random body fluctuation meaning nothing. Third, denial can occur when there is admission that a symptom of disease is present but the gravity of that symptom is discounted; it is evaluated as inconsequential. Fourth, denial can occur when the facts are acknowledged but dismissed as untrue or ill-founded. Finally, denial can occur when there is concurrence that the diagnosis is correct but the consequences from having that disease are ignored.

Denial can only be successful for so long, until symptoms become worse or others push the denier to face reality. But as long as symptoms can remain mild to moderate, someone in denial can remain ensconced in his cocoon, for even years at a time.

TREATMENT CONSIDERATIONS

From the standpoint of CCT, denial is a problem when it is used in the wrong context. In some contexts it has utility. For example, Terry, a dying cancer patient, used denial to live the balance of his life without having to worry about how his life will end. On paper it was clear that his family would absorb a major cut in their standard of living after his death, but he subconsciously chose to believe that everything will be fine for them. While he did what he could to protect them financially, he used denial to avoid worrying about their future, something he could do nothing about. Denial allowed him to face his family's future without dread and anguish. He enjoyed his last days because of self-imposed ignorance.

Once denial is identified, therapists need to discuss with the patient if this is a helpful or harmful strategy, as part of an incentive analysis (Sharoff, 2002). The intent is to discuss any coping strategies in a reflective, objective, fair manner to reduce defensiveness.

One way to deal with denial is by giving the patient specific details about how the body operates when harmful or noncompliant practices occur. Next, ask the patient to take responsibility for engaging in that harmful practice (i.e., Therapist: "Please sign this form, saying, 'I understand that the practice of _____ is harmful to me but I nevertheless plan to pursue that course.' ").

Another way to address denial is by explicating the self-talk that comprises the practice. For instance:

> I will not think about what I am doing or the consequences of my actions. I will believe everything will be okay even though I have been told my behavior will hurt me. As soon as I start feeling better I will tell myself that there is no need to worry about this health problem.

Next, the patient is asked to read his self-talk before engaging in denial, so he is aware of what he is doing. Again, this facilitates responsibility-taking.

A dialogic technique can be used (Hycner, 1985; Polsters, 1973). An adaptive part-of-self is developed to counterbalance the part-of-self engaged in denial. Both the former and the latter are given names (e.g., "my self-caring side versus my hedonistic side"). The healthy part-of-self then talks to the patient before the deleterious practice begins, to avoid the denial practice.

Relapse prevention practice can also work in conjunction with this dialogic technique. A list of high-risk situations are produced that lists where the patient tends to slip, engage in denial, and practice unhealthy actions (Marlatt, 1985). Once on notice that the situation is coming-up, the patient can be watchful for denial and assume the healthy part-of-self beforehand.

REJECTION OF LOSSES STRATEGY

When symptoms first arise, many patients unprepared for the many losses that they will have to endure rise up against the intrusion of disease and reject any more problems in their life. Announcing that they are "damn mad and fed up," they become a combatant against their illness or anyone else who will cause them trouble. Drawing a mental line in the sand, they tell God, fate, health care providers, or their own body, "No more. I have had enough. I will not be penalized by this condition any more." They show irritation and impatience with anyone who frustrates them or causes them to lose anything else, such as time, equanimity, good mood, or further health. A rejection of loss strategy seeks to protect the patient and his family from further injury and adversity caused by disease or treatment. The primary need is safety and security. Grief, frustration, and anger motivate this strategy.

The strategy does have benefit in this regard. By taking a stand, protesting further losses, and airing grievances (overtly or covertly), patients feel more powerful than they actually are. While the presumption of power is illusory, patients feel better when acting as a combatant against a faceless foe. The rejection of losses can even proceed on to real protest, where patients become an advocate for themselves with doctors, insurance companies, or HMOs.

However, problems arise when rejection of losses is used to excess. At this point it often results in noncompliance with the medical regimen if too complicated, and anger and bitterness about the effects of disease. It darkens mood and exacerbates interactions with others, causing patients to feel surly, testy, and cranky. There is often a focus on petty inconveniences in treatment and inordinate time is spent trying to rectify small problems just to show "I won't be pushed around anymore." Often it causes a preoccupation with one's own needs as part of a self-compensation tactic: to give back to oneself after so much has been taken away. The strategy frequently leads to self-pity, to excessively comfort oneself for losses, but this portrays the self as a hapless victim and that results in a sense of powerlessness.

TREATMENT CONSIDERATIONS

Behind the rejection of loss strategy are absolutistic beliefs (e.g., "I will not incur any more losses. Losses should not be happening to me. This is not how my life was supposed to be."). These absolutistic beliefs can be challenged as inflexible and unrealistic. Instead a viewpoint can be promoted that losses will need to be allowed and cannot be ruled out because they are part of the disease process. Therapists can encourage a policy or position that losses are not desirable or not preferable instead of viewing them as awful or the worst. (See next chapter on cognitive restructuring.)

Extensive support will also have to be extended to patients who feel their losses greatly. Time needs to be given to patients to help them to experience their loss and express their feelings about it. Highlighting the flip-side of each feeling is important for a full understanding of the consequences of a loss. If patients express anger then point out the grief and sadness are behind it. If patients are engulfed in sadness, then underscore the rage behind repeated losses. *Constructive mourning* is utilized in this effort (Sharoff, 2004), first to express anger and grief. Then, the intellect is incorporated into a dialogue to provide an objective view of the situation.

Patients need to understand why losses are so troublesome to them. A particular reason is helplessness to avoid further losses. For this problem *helplessness tolerance* and *helplessness accommodation* is useful, to live with losses that cannot be avoided (see chapter 8 and 9, respectively). Losses also result in deprivation, and for that problem the skill of *deprivation allowance* is helpful (Sharoff, 2004).

PRESERVATION STRATEGY

A preservationist strategy seeks to maintain what was good about the premorbid life, which may be lifestyle, career, patterns in relationships, or role activities that supported and helped loved ones. Preservationists do not want to spoil what they had, so they defend against change. Their internal feelings are sadness and frustration, and like the person who rejects losses, they spend considerable time in plaintive contemplation about what was.

Preservationists are different from patients who reject losses in several regards. The former does not engage in protest or bitter denunciations like the latter. Preservationists are not angry or rebellious against conditions or situations that deprive them. Their focus is not on fighting against anything that will cost them further losses. They do not reject their situation as much as they try to keep what they care about going. They expend substantial effort trying to resuscitate or rekindle what was, by fondly remembering a coveted time before the onset of disease, or taking solace in routines that were staples of the old existence.

This is a common strategy of terminally ill patients. For example, when Willard learned that he was dying, he continued to maintain the same patterns he always pursued. He continued to go to work loyally, go to his club activities, frequent his favorite restaurants, etc. He did everything the same way to preserve the life he loved to the very end. Other terminally ill patients practice preservation by working to keep their family at the same standard of living after their death. They do not want their family to have to change anything just because they have died.

This is a common strategy among grieving family members. They keep the home looking the same as when their loved one was alive. They use the deceased's rules and morals to guide their actions ("This is how dad would have done it."). They refuse to date, change habits, or live their life any differently than it was before their spouse died.

TREATMENT CONSIDERATIONS

CCT would treat a preservationist strategy in the initial phase of disease as a time-fit error. In the premorbid days, the tendency to maintain routines and patterns makes life predictable and steady. Doing so organizes existence and forms an appropriate distribution of labor. However, when disease first appears and so much is changing, a preservationist strategy is adopted to forestall change. It is implemented to maintain a world that is slipping away. However, this strategy has a downside and does not fit the needs of the moment. Patients may not be physically able to be their old self. The strategy lulls patients and their significant others into believing everything is okay when that is not the case. It detours everyone from learning coping skills that can aid adjustment. In essence, the strategy is a simplistic, magical answer to a complex problem. There are preferable strategies that can better facilitate adjustment.

However, once the skills that aid adaptation have been learned, the disease has stabilized, and the needs of treatment no longer come first, CCT promotes a preservation strategy. It is most helpful for the time referred to as the consolidation and synthesis phases (see chapter 5). A preservation strategy can encourage the building of a new life style that intertwines elements of the old life. Once a suitable life-style has been established, the strategy maintains routines (e.g., "get up, take my medication, take a walk, have breakfast, etc.").

NORMALIZATION STRATEGY

This is a variation of a preservationist strategy. A patient who practices a normalization strategy dearly seeks a normal life, which is defined as being one's "good old self." Like the preservationist they yearn to maintain the premorbid state, and any change from past ways of being is rejected. Even though medical facts argue for a change in operation and status quo, normalizers fight against that. They want to keep their former life intact.

They are different from the preservationist by what motivates them. The normalizer fears the disease and dreads what lies ahead (e.g., change, deterioration, isolation). The dominant feeling is anxiety. They are scared that their body cannot function like it always has. To cope with this realization, they assiduously work to keep their former self—the premorbid self—intact and running. They desperately seek their old life out of worry that they are not who they used to be. Feeling normal is a dominant need and an end in itself. Meeting others' expectations, maintaining role functioning, and fulfilling established standards—at work or at home—proves to themselves and others "I'm still as good as ever."

To make that point, they force themselves to remain engaged in the same activities they previously pursued, and in fact they often overdo those activities. Habits, routines, and roles are zealously maintained; business as usual is the rule. A demand on self is made to march on at all costs. They continue to take on responsibilities even when the data indicates that less responsibility is required for medical reasons. Facts show that the body cannot handle any more stress but that often fails to persuade them to relinquish activities.

Oppositely, preservationists are not primarily focused on what lies ahead but on what they had in the past. Their dominant feeling is sadness about the loss of the past life. They could accept changes in themselves, and changes in identity forced on them by the disease, if they could preserve their old life and relationships. They do not have anything to prove to others about themselves. They do not fear to be different. They just like what they had and do not want to give it up, just because some disease tells them that it is time to be different.

Normalizers have a set concept of who they should be, and it does not include the identity of someone who has symptoms of disease. Self-concept is based on who they were in the premorbid state, and their intention is to maintain that identity no matter what. They do this to maintain self-esteem. They hate and reject their new self that is dying, disabled, or dysfunctional in any way. They do not like who they have become, and hold the new version of self in contempt.

For example, Ron loved his body, good looks, and personality. He became a great success in everything he ever tried to do. He believed that if he put his mind to something he could do whatever he wanted. He was a walking testimonial to will power. Then a crisis occurred: he developed diabetes. Three times he was hospitalized for doing the same irrational act. He would walk next door to a donut shop and eat one chocolate donut after another until he went into a diabetic coma. Referred to treatment he learned that the diabetes was a narcissistic insult to himself. He could not tolerate the fact that his "perfect body" was now infirm and lacking in some way. Ronald could not allow his diabetes to exist in his body. He set off to show his body who was in charge. Eating one donut after another, he tried to use will power to prove that he could overcome his diabetes and defeat it.

The case of a mastectomy patient illustrates how a normalizer may respond to events as compared to a patient who rejects loss. A normalizer would disapprove of her body because it is no longer "normal" like other woman's bodies. Normalizers would see themselves as no longer being fully equipped. Something vital is missing—their breasts—and in their eyes that makes them a freak. However, following reconstructive surgery, they may feel at peace with themselves because their appearance is back to normal. Patients who pursue rejection of loss will also have a difficult time after a mastectomy, but their focus is on the issue of loss—loss of breasts, loss of identity, or loss of regard from spouse. Their anger focuses on what has been taken from them, and they may even stay focused on this after reconstructive surgery.

TREATMENT CONSIDERATIONS

One way to treat normalizing is to regard it as a coping skills excess. Some of the pursuit is helpful but it is done too much and for too long. It drives medical patients on against the advice of others and ends up hurting their health. The push to be normal is still recommended, but when it becomes counterproductive to medical treatment then the strategy needs to be diminished but not eliminated entirely.

Another way to treat a normalization strategy is by regarding it as a contextualization error. In one context—where disease is not significantly interfering with normal role functioning—a normalization strategy is promoted. At that time, there is a need to avoid focusing on the disease, not talk or complain about physical changes and distress, and return to business as usual. This is a typical strategy for chronic pain patients who have had substantial treatment or surgery and for whom little else medically can be done (Fordyce, 1976; Fordyce & Steger, 1979). They need to return to their previous role functioning as much as possible and sustain old patterns and relationships—without focusing on their symptoms. In another context, where disease has made substantial changes in life functioning and patients cannot return to their premorbid self, a normalization strategy should not be pursued. For example, it could push patients to be someone they are not capable of being due to their symptomatology. It can cause patients to reject adjusting to their disease and learning skills that can facilitate a new way of being, one with less wear and tear on the body.

In one context—in the early phase of disease when treatment and/or surgery is necessary—a normalization strategy can cause patients to be noncompliant and not pursue necessary treatment. That is because treatment indicates that the body and life have to be modified and normalizers do not want to recognize that. In that context, a normalization strategy is discouraged. In another context—in the later phase of disease when further treatment may not be helpful and patients have to return to living with their body as is and adjust to having a disease—a normalization strategy can be helpful and is encouraged. At that time interest in a normal, unfettered existence unaffected by treatment exigencies is beneficial. The strategy can push patients to establish a new identity and routines that will serve as the foundation for a new lifestyle.

The treatment of identity in normalizers is an important matter, because of the degree of distaste of whom the person has become. Their new identity is different from the old one and the old one has been spoiled by disease. Hence, treatment of identity adulteration will be needed. At the same time preserving the premorbid identity as much as possible will be helpful (see chapter 7).

Treatment also has to deal with demands placed on the body to act like its "old self," when that is not possible. Anger at oneself often occurs when expectations cannot be met or standards are not fulfilled. In that case, realistic expectations for the body have to be formed, and *body accommodation* training will be helpful in this effort (Sharoff, 2004). It will coach the patient in how to relate to the body and work with it as a different entity. *Self-support training* will also be quite helpful to maintain a steady, high self-esteem (see chapter 7). Normalizers will put themselves down when the body cannot perform as expected. *Self-boosting* and *self-compassion training* will help to counteract that tendency. A companion skill will also be needed and that is *anger management*. Treatment of arousal and frustration will be important for developing tolerance of the medical condition. *Relaxation training* has a place at that time (see chapter 8).

Because anxiety is high among normalizers, the treatment of anxiety will become paramount in order to overcome the feeling of crisis. The first treatment task is to bring attention to the fact that behind the patient's need to be normal is a basic fear of being different. *Acceptance training* is needed to ease self-rejection. Next, the patient needs to be taught *anxiety tolerance* skills such as *relaxation, self-monitoring, sensory-diversion,* and self-instruction training (see chapter 8). This will make life more comfortable psychologically. It will also develop self-assurance that the self can manage its situation. Normalizers need to know that they know how to cope, and that will decrease fear about the disease. At the same time they need to know that their anxiety about their well-being will not go away because their functioning is being challenged daily. This will require the skill of *anxiety accommodation* (Sharoff, 2004). Another reason for anxiety is uncertainty. For that problem, *uncertainty tolerance* will be helpful along with *optimism training* (Sharoff, 2004); included in this is the practice of *bright-side thinking* (Sharoff, 2002, 2004).

SELF-NUMBING STRATEGY

This coping skill is practiced secondarily to an awareness about the effects of disease. Feeling psychological pain from the many changes in their life, some patients seek to evade that pain by numbing themselves. They do not want to face the fact that life is going to end, be substantially different, or will entail significant suffering. They evade reality by dulling awareness of who they have become and what they are experiencing. By numbing their senses about who they are they remove themselves from a disappointing life.

Self-numbing can be practiced in several ways. A common way is abuse of alcohol, prescription analgesics, or street drugs. Another method is overeating, where food is used as a tranquilizer for anxiety. Depression can also be used as a form of self-numbing when one becomes psychologically disengaged. There can be withdrawal from the world by excessive sleep or depression. Others numb themselves by engaging in nonstop activities or being a workaholic; if they are busy enough then they do not have to feel their emotions. A final method of self-numbing is staying in a state of shock upon hearing one's medical diagnosis.

The problem with self-numbing is that it works. Patients use it instead of learning more beneficial ways of coping that can facilitate adjustment, such as acceptance and tolerance abilities. It is a quick way out of dilemmas and has benefit as long as it is practiced. But when the form of numbing wears off (e.g., the patient sobers up), the pain from disease returns, and at that time anxiety is felt about "what is happening to me?"

TREATMENT CONSIDERATIONS

One way to treat self-numbing is by dealing with it as a coping skills excess. That is, a prudent amount of self-numbing tactics can be adaptive and beneficial. Certainly included in this effort is the taking of prescription drugs according to medical recommendations. The consumption of a glass of wine at dinner (if medically supported) to quell stress, and regular napping can be beneficial. Escaping into enjoyable sensory activities is a type of self-numbing, such as by taking a hot bath at the end of the day.

When self-numbing is used to excess, it can produce a dual diagnosis of alcohol and/or drug addiction along with the adjustment disorder of not coping with the disease. It often produces other disorders such as depression or marital maladjustment. In that case, providers need to be versed in substance abuse treatment and marital counseling.

A dominant reason self-numbing is practiced is because of rejection of suffering. The self-number does not want to face life with pain or distress. *Assimilation of suffering* will be needed for that problem (see chapter 6; Sharoff, 2004). That will prepare the patient for a life that cannot avoid suffering.

SELF-DESTRUCTION STRATEGY

Self-destruction is a maladaptive coping strategy that develops due to depression about the body and lifestyle as a consequence of disease. It is formed as a result of an inability to adjust to the realities of existence. While calling it a coping strategy sounds self-contradictory, it nevertheless provides patients with a means to manage their emotions. It offers an outlet for rage by destroying the sick body. Revenge against the body for becoming sick then has an outlet in self-destruction. Revenge against significant others can be practiced by hurting the self, which causes others to worry. Anger at life or God can be displaced against the body.

Self-destruction can occur in several ways. One method is by using alcohol or drugs to excess. Another method is by driving the body incessantly to punish it, such as by working long hours. A third method is noncompliance with the medical regimen, which in turn causes symptoms to flare up in the body. Other methods include reckless driving, becoming accident prone, and suicide.

TREATMENT CONSIDERATIONS

The self-destructive patient refuses to live life with a chronic or terminal illness. These patients are not aware or are in denial that they are self-destructive. Their actions have to be interpreted as such to forge realization of intent. The cause of self-destruction is often a rejection of suffering, and for that problem the skill of *assimilation of suffering* needs to be practiced (chapter 6). Disliking life because it is so physically unpleasant, patients unconsciously turn to self-destruction to escape from life. For that problem, they need to know *amelioration of discomfort* tactics, to ease physical distress and pain and to coexist with their disease (Sharoff, 2004).

A primary reason for self-destruction is anathema toward oneself. There is often irrational, unreasonable thinking behind self-hatred and that has to be explored. Patients often blame themselves for becoming ill. To treat this problem, *forgiveness training* is helpful (Sharoff, 2002). Once patients soften their dislike toward themselves, *self-boosting* can be initiated to find positive ways to see oneself (chapter 7).

With self-destructive patients, risk of suicide has to be assessed. If need be, a contract for safety can be utilized and put in effect until the patient realizes that a meaningful life can be achieved, given the parameters imposed by the disease. The activity of *meaning-making* will be quite helpful for this purpose (Sharoff, 2004). *Problem solving* will also be beneficial to show patients how to solve their problems without having to resort to suicide.

Many self-destructive patients are simply overwhelmed by the sheer number of disappointments caused by their disease. To help with this matter, *disappointment tolerance* and *disappointment accommodation* are useful (Sharoff, 2004). They will help patients accept their situation and face up to it, instead of seeking escape through self-harm.

DISSOLUTION

There is a variant of the self-destruction strategy—a dissolution strategy. It involves destruction of who the patient was in the premorbid state. It is announced by the call, "I just don't care any more," and with that the patient wipes away former goals, habits, patterns, roles, or lifestyle. Central to the strategy of dissolution is a disqualification of the former life plan. The intention is to no longer play by the old rules or comply with old policies.

Anything can replace the premorbid self. The patient enters a life in schism, where any fragment or part-of-self can become dominant, select the goals for the future, and guide decision making. This is a type of decomposition and reformulation of the self. Dissolution can be a temporary or permanent way of living. As a temporary phenomena, new policies, goals, or roles come into effect for a while and then are replaced by another part of self that seizes control and adopts another plan. As a permanent solution a new lifestyle replaces the old one and stays in effect.

To offer examples of a dissolution strategy, there is the person who quits a long held job and career plan and takes a "fun job" that she always wanted to do. There is the patient who decides to drop everything and become a traveler, taking trips to places he always dreamed of visiting. Other patients decide to have one or more affairs, to break away from the constraints of marriage and sexually experiment. Others decide to become a "hippie" and experiment with alternative lifestyles, which often involves drugs. The dissolution strategy is commonly seen in terminally ill patients who "don't give a damn anymore" and instead pursue a life more controlled by caprice, the desire to rebel, and hidden longings. In each case patients give themselves permission to vary their pattern and allow a hidden or suppressed part-of-self to emerge and become dominant. Other parts-of-self are submerged as the new dominant part makes life decisions.

TREATMENT CONSIDERATIONS

The dissolution strategy emerges because disease has such a major impact on people. It makes people realize that life is short and fleeting, and that there is not sufficient time left to follow old scripts anymore. Dissolution patients want to grab hold of their existence, do what is meaningful, and live life one day at a time. This is the beneficial side to this strategy and treatment needs to support that effort.

The job of the therapist is to act as an overseer, so dissolution occurs in a reasonable, prudent manner. This is accomplished when there is an integration of the various parts of self. Integration avoids the abrupt switching to other pursuits, which can be quite shocking to significant others in the patient's life. It overcomes the problem of giving one part of self too much of a voice and power over future decision making while limiting the influence of other parts. To facilitate integration, the various parts of self are identified and each part's desires and needs are heard. The intellect then reflects on which way to proceed, so a course of action is taken in an orderly, consistent fashion. This way the total interests of the person are well represented and pursued but not impulsively so.

The downside to dissolution is noncompliance with the medical regimen. Stung by loss of control due to the disease, dissolution patients often rebel against being controlled by anyone or anything, such as medical requirements. If in recovery, a patient may resume drinking or drugging again. If he used to exercise regularly, he may decide to lead a slothful, lazy existence. Treatment needs to explicate the internal dialogue behind dissolution (e.g., "I will only do what feels good now, because I do not know how much longer I have to live."), so patients know how shortsighted the strategy can be. A healthy part of self can be commissioned to counteract the impulsive part of self (e.g., "Don't live for the moment, and then hurt the future by acting imprudently."). Cognitive restructuring can also be done with a part-of-self, examining its thinking for rationality (see chapter 4).

SUMMARY

There are several types of maladaptive strategies of which providers need to be aware. A denial strategy pushes important knowledge of the disease out of consciousness. A rejection of loss strategy refuses to live with losses mandated by the disease. A preservation strategy wants to hide in premorbid routines instead of making an adjustment to live with the disease. A normalization strategy does the same because there is fright about the future. A self-numbing strategy wants to dull awareness of what life has become. A self-destructive strategy seeks self-harm to a body that has become ill. A dissolution strategy seeks an end to a former lifestyle and the emergence of a more meaningful course of action, but often it is taken against common sense and medical advice.

Chapter 4

The Cognitive Restructuring Option

Coping skills therapy is part of cognitive behavioral therapy (CBT). From its first appearance in the 1960's (Beck, 1963; Ellis, 1962), CBT has achieved a major standing in the field of psychotherapy (Dobson, 1988, 2001). (See Dobson and Block (1988) for review.) It has been referred to as a "paradigm revolution" (Mahoney, 1974). CBT is comprised of cognitive restructuring and coping skills therapy. Without question, the dominant approach in CBT is cognitive restructuring (CR). This chapter will present the practice theory and methodology of CR. It will give examples of how it operates and some of its dominant or most common techniques. And finally, the chapter includes the drawbacks of this approach with medical patients.

PRACTICE THEORY

The basic principal behind the cognitive restructuring approach is that cognition mediates between stimulus and response, and that people will change their behavior when they change their cognition. Cognitive restructuring rests on the theory that appraisals and perceptions of events affect the response to an event, and that behavior change will follow a change in thinking (Beck, 1976; Beck, Rush, Shaw, & Emery, 1979; Ellis, 1971).

The practice theory states that irrational, unrealistic, or maladaptive thinking lies behind pathology. Invalid, illogical, or inappropriate thoughts about the activating event and not the event itself account for more of the disturbance. By assessing cognitive activity and then changing it to become rational, realistic, or adaptive, people can resolve affective and behavioral problems. Cognitive activity can include cognitive content, such as core irrational beliefs (Ellis & Harper, 1975) or cognitive distortions, which are mechanisms that occur in the process of thinking that lead to unrealistic beliefs (Beck et al., 1979; Burns, 1980; Dryden & Ellis, 1988).

There are two models of CR. One model is termed the rationalist approach, representing the work of Ellis (1962, 1971; Ellis & Grieger, 1977; Ellis & MacLaren, 1998), Beck (1976; Beck et al., 1979; Beck & Emery, 1988; Beck, Freeman, & Associates, 1990), and Meichenbaum (1977, 1985). The second model is termed the constructivist approach, representing the work of Kelly (1991), Guidano (1988), Mahoney (1977, 1995), Neimeyer (1985), and others. (For an excellent discussion of the differences between these two approaches, see Mahoney 1988.) The rationalists have popularized cognitive restructuring with a concise, clear, easy to implement, sharply focused protocol that most therapists identify as THE model for changing thinking. Because the dominant cognitive restructuring approach is the rationalist model, this book will focus on how it would be used with medical patients.

METHODOLOGY OF COGNITIVE RESTRUCTURING

Below are the steps for restructuring cognition elucidated by cognitive therapy (Beck et al., 1979).

1) Identify the activating event that is of concern to a person.
2) Identify the response of the person to the event, including the emotional, physiological, and behavioral levels of the response.
3) Identify the beliefs about that activating event and the response to that event.

3a) Inquire how certain that person is that his/her belief is realistic, rational, and adaptive, from zero to one hundred, with one hundred being total certainty that a belief is correct.

4) Convert the belief into a hypothesis that can be tested. The belief that was taken for granted as a fact is then scrutinized in a scientific investigation.

4a) Have the patient adopt an objective stance by being willing to examine their thinking dispassionately, instead of automatically adopting it as valid.

5) Collect evidence about the event to confirm or reject the hypothesis. Challenge and counter the patient's thinking so it is examined critically.

5a) Another option is proposing alternative perspectives, such as alternative meanings for the data, alternative consequences in addition to the patient's presumed consequence, alternative causal events besides the patient's presumed cause of the situation.

6) When enough data is collected, inquire if the hypothesis is correct.

7) If the hypothesis is rejected, develop new thinking to substitute for it that is rational, realistic, and adaptive.

8) Gain acceptance of the new thinking. Show the patient that it leads to less negative feeling, less physiological disturbance, and more constructive behavior.

Rational-Emotive-Behavioral Therapy (REBT)'s approach is quite similar to that of cognitive therapy. The differences between the two are in part stylistic. REBT operates in a more polemical and confrontative manner with patients (Ellis & MacLaren, 1998; Wessler & Wessler, 1980). When it counters patient thinking it calls it "disputation." Cognitive therapy seeks to develop a collegial relationship with patients as both work to discover what the facts are. There are also differences in emphasis. REBT focuses more on absolutistic thinking while cognitive therapy focuses on inaccurate, unrealistic perceptions.

TYPES OF BELIEFS

There are common beliefs that CR works with routinely, and they are considered the dominant cause of pathology. Sharoff (2002) maintains faith in those beliefs—what he refers to as "certainistic thinking"—is the dominant cause of pathology. That is because patients are certain their thinking is correct and remain true believers.

ABSOLUTISTIC THINKING

This is a normative belief that sets a rigid, unbending, unyielding rule or standard for a person, place, group, higher power, or event (Dryden & Ellis, 1988, 2001). The belief is a demand or command that there must be total, unconditional adherence to a rule or standard with no exceptions. Inherent in the belief is the idea that compliance with the rule or standard is imperative, vital, and of the utmost importance. The absolutistic thought will strongly influence the evaluation of the situation if the rule is broken or the standard is not met, resulting in a severe, extreme evaluation such as "awful" or "terrible." Ellis (Dryden & Ellis, 1988, 2001) has stated that absolutistic thinking is the dominant cause of pathology.

In general, disputes for absolutistic thinking have the following therapeutic intentions:

a) Change the viewpoint that consequences from not following a demand or rule will not be awful but unpleasant or unwanted

b) Change the evaluation of the event so it is less extreme and more reasonable, to think in terms of undesirable or unfortunate.

c) Create willingness to believe that not following a rule or living up to a standard is not awful but a non-preferable situation.

d) Challenge the underlying philosophy and rigid rules that cause someone to respond as they do.

UNREALISTIC THINKING

There can be unrealistic thinking about what a situation means, about what will happen in the future, and how one situation can affect another. A thought about what something means deals with the definition of the situation. Thoughts about the future deal with predictions or probability judgments. Thoughts about one situation leading to another can be catastrophic thinking.

A. Unrealistic Judgments about Meaning

This is an incorrect judgment about the definition of a situation, based on an inaccurate reading of the facts. Empirical evidence does not support that conclusion, or the so-called data is unreliable or invalid (Beck et al., 1979; Salkovskis, 1996).

Disputes about meaning have the following therapeutic intentions:

a) Secure evidence to support a supposed fact (How do you know X is the case?).
b) Show that a belief is only a hypothesis that cannot be taken for granted as the truth without investigating the facts. Create a tendency in patients to scientifically examine their conclusions about meaning.
c) Demonstrate that there is not just one correct meaning proposition for a situation to decrease faith in certainistic thinking.
d) Secure an objective, sensible definition of a concept or situation.

B. Inaccurate Predictions

This is an incorrect probability judgment or prediction because it is not sufficiently based on data. Someone believes that there is a high probability that something will happen in the future when in actuality there is a much lower probability of that occurring. The prediction is a presumption that something will occur, but it is largely unsupported by data. Catastrophic thinking is a type of prediction supported by other predictions leading to an undesirable outcome.

Disputes about predictions have the following therapeutic intentions:

a) Show that a prediction is not supported by enough facts, to reduce loyalty to it.
b) Show that that there are other consequences besides the one the patient believes will happen.
c) Reveal that one incorrect assumption is used as the foundation for other incorrect assumptions, to show that the future does not have to be as bleak as presumed by the patient.

EXTREME, SEVERE EVALUATIVE JUDGMENTS

This is a judgment that attempts to fix or establish the worth of something or someone, but the evaluation is too extreme and severe. An example is a judgment that declares something is awful, terrible, horrible, or the worst, when it is not that way. The evaluation rates something's degree of "badness" incorrectly and does not take into consideration other events that are worse. The tendency to do this is referred to as *awfulizing* (Dryden & Ellis, 1988). To treat this problem, therapists can compare the patient's situation to others to assess which is worse. This facilitates objectivity and more reasonable ratings.

ATTRIBUTION ERROR

This is a conclusion about cause and effect. An attribution error can be made in two different ways. There is a presumption that something internal to the individual has caused a problem when external factors are to blame as well. Or, there is a presumption that something external to the individual has caused a problem when internal factors within a person are to blame as well. Too much weight is given to an internal or external cause, and other factors are not considered. To treat this problem, therapists need to show that causality is complex and that there are multiple causes for events when casting blame.

REDUCTIONISTIC THINKING

This is a belief that a complex whole with many attributes is actually composed of only one or a few attributes. An event or person is then equated to that small, limited group of attributes, which becomes salient when perceiving the self and dominates thinking. To treat this problem, therapists need to demonstrate the complexity of the self to illustrate that only a few prototypical features are being used to define it.

MALADAPTIVE AND NON-UTILITARIAN THINKING

This is a belief that harms adaptation, or prevents or hinders a desired outcome from occurring. To treat this problem, therapists need to demonstrate that what people think is instrumental and affects their chances of achieving an outcome. Therapists need to show that thoughts can aid or hinder goal attainment.

TREATMENT FOR DISALLOWANCE OF DISEASE

Having explained the technique of cognitive restructuring and what it seeks to correct, let us now examine how it would be applied to treat a crucial, maladaptive coping strategy—disallowance of disease. The beliefs that form that strategy are the focus of attention.

Disallowance of disease is a major problem in health care. It is a policy about illness, where it is rejected along with the effect disease has on the patient and his or her family. Intellectually, patients may recognize that they have a disease and that it will be manifested in various ways. Emotionally, though, there is a refusal to accept that fact. Or, there is acceptance of the diagnosis but not the symptoms of the disease ("I know I have chronic fatigue but I hate feeling tired all the time."). This is not denial but conscious protest and rejection of the condition. On an emotional level there is disgust, antagonism, and hate. That hatred can be discharged against the patient's body, where it is viewed in a derisive, demeaning way. The hatred can be discharged against the disease, where it becomes an external entity or object invading the body that receives scorn and derision ("This stinking disease. It is miserable."). Overall, there is an unwillingness to tolerate and accommodate to the presence of disease because the patient wants it out of his or her body and life.

There are five beliefs that underpin the disallowance of disease. Following is an examination of how CR would deal with those beliefs, and a comparison of how a coping skills approach would deal with the belief.

1.   This disease shouldn't be happening to me. My life should not be disease-ridden. **I want this illness out of my life.**

This belief states the patient's policy or position (in italics) on his or her medical condition. Patients may or may not verbalize the above policy openly, but their degree of consternation and chagrin indicates disallowance of disease, revealed as dissatisfaction and protest about being ill and suffering through the consequences from being that way.

Cognitive restructuring asserts that behind this belief is a philosophy not to be limited and left powerless by forces greater than oneself. The philosophy propels the person to assiduously combat those forces and self-righteously take a stand against a situation perceived as unjust. In such a case CR would seek to make a *philosophical shift* in the patient (McMullin, 1986), asserting that a core epistemological mistake has been made to overcome a situation and transcend one's limited, helpless capacity when that is not possible. The treatment goal is to change the patients' philosophy to accept powerlessness when it is forced on them by invisible super-forces (e.g., disease, HMOs). Instead, a new philosophy is stressed to only take a reasonable, prudent position on the situation where patients state their preference: "I do not like what is happening to me."

In general, CR pays special attention to the absolutistic nature of the policy belief in statement number one ("This disease SHOULD NOT be happening to me."). The belief implicitly, categorically demands that the disease, God, fate, fortune, or medical providers must change the situation. In essence, the belief makes a demand for an exclusion from harm: "I should not be penalized or put at a disadvantage by this disease." Hence, behind the disallowance of disease is a claim for **special person status**, which the disease, God, fate, or fortune does not confer on the individual.

The overriding mission of CR is to change the policy belief. One technique for doing this is by using a forced perceptual shift technique (Ellis & Harper, 1975; McMullin, 1986). Patients are given two policy beliefs side-by-side to one another and then select the one that causes the *least* harm. First, the patient's own irrational demand for exclusion from disease is presented. Next, an alternative policy is stated that shuns demandingness: "I wish this disease was not happening to me. I wish this disease would cause me fewer problems. I really want it to disappear." By thinking this way, patients only make requests of forces greater than the self, which is an appropriate, reasonable, rational response to determined events. This type of thinking does not exaggerate unfortunate events by typifying them as awful or the worst thing that could ever have happened to them. It avoids catastrophizing. It results in a lower level of negative emotion that is more tolerable, where someone feels exceptionally sad and grieves but does not feel enraged or depressed. Patients say each statement out loud and then experience the affect of each thought on their feelings. They then select which will cause the least negative emotion, which obviously would be the second statement.

CCT would emphasize different matters than CR. CCT theorizes that when CR focuses on the idea of preference as much as it does (e.g., "I want this disease to disappear."), it inadvertently maintains the protest against disease, but at a milder level. This continues the disallowance of disease. It also keeps the disease in the foreground of the mind. Instead, CCT would seek integration of the disease into the patient's life, trying to make it another facet of the individual (albeit a major feature). Instead of focusing on responding to the symptoms of disease as unfortunate or undesirable, CCT would emphasize **assimilation of suffering**, where suffering becomes an unwanted but normal part of a medical patient's existence. This has the benefit of gradually moving the disease into the background of the mind, where it does impact situations but is not the dominant, foreground issue.

CCT would not primarily focus on the policy belief but instead emphasizes the executive beliefs, which would direct the patient to tolerate the disease. CCT agrees with the CR position that people in general would feel better with a milder policy belief ("I prefer not having this disease."). But if the patient still feels strongly opposed to his or her disease that is not disputed. Instead, *the focus shifts to* **coping with the prevailing reality** *of the moment.*

By doing so, patients would not be so troubled by the consequences of their disease and irrational policy belief. They would not feel such a need to disallow and protest against their condition.

2. My disease causes me a great deal of distress and aggravation. I have been penalized greatly by it. I have had to endure many disappointments and have been deprived in so many ways. ***I'm fed up. I hate this situation I am in.***

This belief reveals the response to the consequences from having a disease. The first part of the statement describes the activating event (the accumulation of distress, penalties, etc.) and the second part is the response to it (in bold type). The response includes hatred and exasperation.

A common intervention in cognitive therapy is to question if the description of the activating event (in this case the activating event is the consequences from having a disease) is an accurate portrayal of the facts. That is, is the situation as bad as the patient believes it is? Has there been as many disappointments or as much deprivation as the patient believes there has been? An inaccurate characterization of the situation results in an unrealistic meaning about it (e.g., "This is an awful situation I am in."). That will motivate the response to disallow the disease. To gauge the accuracy of the belief, a cognitive therapist (Beck et al., 1979) will convert the descriptive judgement into a hypothesis ("Is it true that your disease has caused you as much trouble as you say it has?"). Data will be collected to make that determination.

If the description of the activating event is accurate, then the next issue that needs to be examined is the patient's response: ***is the hatred of disease and the consequences from having it rational and adaptive?*** REBT (Ellis & Abrams, 1994) has no problem with a patient hating their disease. The following statement is labeled sensible and rational, "I really hate being afflicted with this condition . . . how sad and obnoxious it is! I strongly wish that it would disappear. . . . " (p. 47). Hatred—a strong feeling—is not addressed and treated in REBT as long as the patient thinks rationally, when he prefers but does not demand that the disease disappear. That is considered adaptive.

CCT agrees with REBT that the above belief is rational. It will decrease negative emotion and in the short-term that is adaptive. In the long-term, though, maintaining anger and feeling hatred toward the disease is not adaptive. The hatred reveals disallowance of the disease, and that response is non-utilitarian. Feeling hatred easily leads to an overall feeling of dissatisfaction, greater agitation, bitterness, and depression. Oppositely, *a utilitarian response **accepts and integrates** the disease into one's life (because that is the reality the patient has to live with), co-exists with disease gracefully and peacefully, and does not begrudge anyone—oneself, God, or others—for causing it.* Thus, CCT encourages providers to help patients integrate their disease into their life. Hatred obstructs that process. It shows and perpetuates unwillingness to adjust and accommodate to the inevitability of the consequences from disease, which often includes disappointment, deprivation, frustration, distress, penalties, and disadvantage. Hence, when CCT detects hatred of disease, it works to induct patients into using skills that accommodate negative emotions when they cannot be avoided. Once patients learn to live with those emotions, hatred of the disease decreases.

*3.   This disease has caused me enough problems. **I refuse to accept anymore discomfort, disappointment, and deprivation.***

This belief takes a position on the consequences of having disease. When overpowering forces like contagion and aging usurp control from the individual, so many respond by irrationally trying to limit the damage that disease, treatment, or aging cause. Overcome with rage about being impotent, a policy is formulated (in bold italics) to take charge of their life again. Mentally, patients tell disease, God, or medical personnel, "No more." Some medical patients will openly say, "I've had enough," while others keep this thought to themselves because it sounds irrational to make demands on God or a pathology. People's reactions—irritability, frustration, outrage—reveals the presence of this policy.

Once patients concur that this is how they think, CR would deal with this belief as an unrealistic, wishful thought to avoid anymore penalty and disadvantage. However, medical patients' chagrin and consternation about their health problems reveal a much more profound problem, an attempt to disallow defining features of the disease.

That is, if someone has a disease that normally, routinely results in hassle, disappointment, deprivation, and discomfort that is a relevant, prototypical feature of the concept (in this case the concept being that particular disease). If so, then those features are part of the category; they come with the package and have to be accepted as what will be. *Maladjustment occurs when medical patients become upset that defining features of a concept exist.* Anger about the consequences from having a disease shows rejection of the defining features of that category.

It is human, though, to hate troublesome, unpleasant, unwanted, undesirable features of a concept (in this case disease or the treatment for disease). Yet, CCT would not consider that a rational response. If someone knows about the features of a concept (e.g., the nature of a person) but still becomes upset that the concept has that feature then that does not make sense. *"Coming to terms" with something means adjusting to the relevant, prototypical features of the concept (Rosch, 1973, 1975; Rosch & Mervis, 1975; Rosch, Mervis, Gray, Johnson, & Boyes-Braem, 1976).* In the case of disease, the features are disappointment, deprivation, etc.

Providers need to help patients accept the features that comes with their disease, the features of a concept and their relationship to one another. All features of a concept interrelate. For instance, a certain pathogen has attacked the neurological system of a patient causing her not to be able to ambulate properly, which in turn makes walking much more difficult. This means that there will be more frustration in her life due to the demyelination of the white matter of her brain and spinal cord. Hence, increased frustration and central nervous system pathology are interrelated features of her disease. If she is to progress, she needs to be engaged in the activity of *"**feature learning**,"* which is the act of learning about a concept—in this case multiple sclerosis (MS)—and the relationship among the relevant features that define the concept. Each feature is inextricably intertwined with other ones because they share a relationship. One cannot be cleaved from the other. If a person has one feature (e.g., demyelination) then she is stuck with other features (frustration) as well.

Problems begin when people seek to select the features of the concept that they are willing to co-exist with and reject those that are deemed undesirable. They remain unwilling to allow and accept all relevant features of the concept. They form a policy that demands that certain prototypical features of the category—in this case MS—should not be part of the mix. That underlying irrational belief is a major reason for maladjustment to disease.

Cognitive restructuring would treat this problem by helping the medical patient to adopt a rational response to unwanted, prototypical features of the category. Essentially, it encourages the patient to think, "Having this dominant feature of the category is undesirable and unfortunate, but I am powerless to eliminate that feature that defines the category." CR would identify the concept and the features of it ("You have a disease that will cause routine deprivation.") and help the patient adjust to that reality. Socratic questioning (Ellis & Bernard, 1985) could be used in this effort, where questions are posed to the patient to allow him or her to discover a rational position ("You may not like a feature of your disease but can you eliminate it?").

CCT would deal with the refusal to endure anymore negative consequences from disease by discussing the need for ***assimilation of suffering***. It would refer to the rejection of negative consequences as a rejection of further suffering. The feelings behind that position—frustration, fear, helplessness—are then discussed to show their influence in forming the policy to reject negative consequences. This would lead to the induction into assimilation of suffering (see Sharoff, 2004, for fuller discussion).

CCT would also separate the behavioral response to negative consequences from the internal response. It would encourage patients to fight—on a behavioral level only—to change their situation, so they are not as deprived or disappointed as they are. At the same time CCT would encourage an internal response that discourages the battle against the prevailing reality of the moment, which may be deprivation, disappointment, or whatever. It would encourage internal ***accommodation*** to the prevailing reality, because that is what exists at that moment in time and must be accepted. Three skills especially would be proposed to help that effort: ***disappointment accommodation*** training, ***deprivation allowance*** training, and ***helplessness tolerance***. Either directly (through self-instruction training self-dialogue) or indirectly (through such tactics as imagery, symbolic gesturing, or other measures discussed in the Coping Skills Book), these skills would alter the absolutistic belief, "I must not be harmed by this disease."

4. This disease is awful. My life has been awful since I got this disease.

Medical patients quite commonly evaluate their disease and its effects as awful, terrible, horrible, or "the worst." The rating casts the situation in a dark, gloomy light, causing more intense, negative feeling. CR asserts that no medical situation is awful and nothing makes it terrible. "Awful means 100% bad or as bad as it could possibly be. But just about nothing is 100% bad, as it could always be even worse than it is," according to Ellis and Abrams (1994, p. 56). They maintain that even a 99% bad situation could still be worse; there could be even more pain, more deprivation, etc. They assert that even a fatal ailment is not awful (Ellis & Abrams, 1994). It is only very, very bad. A death may be called catastrophic by the patient, because it ends his/her life, but things could always be worse, if not for the patient then his family.

In working with medical patients, this argument is advanced using *objective countering* (McMullin, 1986). Questions are posed that help patients weigh one situation against other ones. This is termed "*relativistic thinking*," where an activating event is viewed relative to another when determining how bad each one is. This creates a broader perspective, that the disease is not the worst thing that could have befallen someone. Essentially, this is a "count your blessings" idea: be grateful for what you have because you could have even less. Supposedly, this perspective will lighten the patient's load (see below for CCT's position on this viewpoint). CR can also use a semantic intervention (Wessler & Wessler, 1980), where other words (e.g., unwanted, non-preferable) are substituted for the severe, extreme rating, and patients then note the affect this has on their emotions. Language is analyzed regarding its effect on outcome.

5. I cannot bear having this disease (or my symptoms, or my treatment). I cannot stand what is happening to my life.

This belief addresses the internal problem of tolerating something that is difficult, distressing, or discomforting. One way to treat this belief is by dealing with it as an unrealistic assessment. Cognitive therapy

(Beck et al., 1979) would convert the thought into a hypothesis and collect data to determine if the patient is truly unable to tolerate difficult, hard times. Patients' histories are reviewed, and from that some situations are selected to demonstrate that they do have an ability to bear-up and cope, even in hard times.

There are other disputation techniques for this belief. Exaggeration can be tried, where the patient's supposed inability is enlarged (McMullin, 1986). "Is it true that you are completely, totally unable to manage in this tough time. Are you correct that you simply lack all of what it takes to handle this difficult situation?" Another option is a *method of difference* technique (McMullin, 1986). This approach identifies the same situation where different outcomes have occurred but shows that different outcomes are due to different beliefs about the situation.

Many patients, though, are correct when they say that they cannot tolerate their disease and that is why they disallow it. They have realistically appraised their abilities and find that they lack coping capacity. In this case the problem does not lie with the patient's thinking but with a coping skills deficit.

PROBLEMS WITH THE CR MODEL

Having presented the cognitive restructuring model, let us now look at it critically, regarding its role in health care. It certainly does offer a powerful approach that can be uplifting and efficacious. However, the approach also has its limitations.

First, we will appraise the idea of CR that any disease is not awful, just undesirable. This message can be uplifting to patients who have a nonsymptomatic disease and/or one that causes only mild to moderate injury, disability, and discomfort. However, the message to think relativistically (compare one's plight to others who have it worse) is often greeted by resistance if not disdain by those who have a severely painful condition, or a crippling, disabling, or terminal disease. Telling a terminal illness patient that his or her life-ending disease is not awful or terrible—just non-preferable—will be viewed as ridiculous and hallow. Telling that patient to take solace that worse things could have occurred is of little consolation. While CR wants medical patients to embrace objective reality, they often stay mired in their subjective point-of-view. Treatment at this point can break down over the matter of quantity: how bad is the patient's plight—awful or just very, very bad.

CCT, on the other hand, sees no harm in agreeing with the patient's extreme, severe evaluation of their situation. It does not believe that treatment has to be harmed by validating the conceptualization that the patient's ordeal is awful, as long as he employs needed coping skills. The problem is not with the irrational, unrealistic evaluation but with the inability or unwillingness to cope with the situation. CCT agrees with CR that awfulizing is not rational or realistic, and can lead to a melancholy state or self-pity. However, *rationality is not necessarily isomorphic to adaptation,* as Meichenbaum (1977) points out. Rationality is not a cure-all or salvation alone. People can be irrational but as long as they practice skills leading to adaptation then their thinking (including their policy beliefs) does not have to be toxic or *that* problematic. Again, this is a quantitative issue. Irrational thinking like awfulizing causes some degree of disturbance, but far more disturbance is caused by irrational, maladaptive coping strategies and other unhealthy combinations of skills, coping skills deficits, skills used to excess, and skills used in the wrong context, in the wrong time, or sequence.

Cognitive restructuring technique results in another problem with medical patients and also the bereaved. It is not with the content of the message but how it is delivered. CR has a style that may not appeal to a certain type of patient. The crisp, direct, cerebral, disputational nature of the rationalist approach can be interpreted as uncaring and unfeeling by patients desiring a therapist who is "softer," emotionally-oriented, and non-confrontive. Martin and Doka (2000) have identified one type of patient they term "intuitive," and they need to emote and cry, gain support from others, and need to be aware of and in touch with their feelings, especially when beset by grief. They seek a therapist who will spend considerable time helping them experience and express their feelings while validating their subjective worldview ("You really are in a rough situation. This has been dreadful for you!"). The CR format and style does not lend itself to the needs of such a patient. Staying on a cognitive level with such a patient risks a break in rapport that can result in rejection of treatment or therapist.

The therapist practicing CR tries to stay on a cerebral level in the hope that patients will be converted to operating on that level as well. However, before medical patients can become cognitively oriented, they may have a need to discharge some of their emotion via catharsis and ventilation, but CR does not encourage that at all! CCT concedes that medical patients and the bereaved are often impacted with emotion, so they can greatly benefit from the cool, dispassionate, cognitive orientation of CR. It can help them sort out their emotions, and help them understand why they feel so intensely about certain matters. Before this can occur, though, *therapists need to modify the therapeutic style of CR with medical patients.* More time needs to be spent on their emotional needs, including the acknowledgement of their suffering, losses, predicaments, conflicts, and dilemmas. Medical patients need to feel that the health provider feels their pain and understands their ordeal. Far more time needs to be given for emotional support. A caring, empathic, feeling-oriented way of operating needs to occur as a transition into cognitive examination. Relationship is crucial in working with medical patients and the bereaved, and that relationship is *initially* build not on the shoulders of cognitive analysis but on the heart of a feeling-oriented provider who appears to be understanding and supportive.

SUMMARY

Cognitive restructuring maintains that the belief about the activating event is the primary reason for pathology. It works to change thinking that is irrational, unrealistic, or maladaptive. It uses various techniques to change excessive confidence in the accuracy of a belief, that CCT terms certainistic thinking. It focuses on certain kinds of thoughts: absolutistic thinking, unrealistic thinking (which includes unrealistic judgments about meaning, inaccurate predictions, and catastrophic thinking), extreme, severe evaluative judgments, attribution errors, reductionistic thinking, and maladaptive thinking. To assess how CR operates, the maladaptive coping strategy of disallowance of disease is examined.

Chapter 5

Assessment of Adjustment

The impact of disease is related to how well people adjust to it. A good adjustment overrides the pernicious affects of disease. The disease exists but the injury from it is minimal. The disease does not cause the patient to feel abnormal, even though the body is abnormal. There is satisfaction about various matters, although the person's overall situation is far from satisfying. Oppositely, a poor adjustment makes the disease far more oppressive. There may be minimal disease effects but extensive life effects (e.g., decrement in role maintenance, abandonment of activity pursuits). Symptoms may become overwhelming even with minimal anatomical damage. The role of medical patient dominates identity.

Hence, adjustment to disease is a crucial variable in the over all treatment of chronic and terminal illness. Knowing how well patients adjust is an important consideration, to determine what needs to be addressed in therapy. This chapter presents assessment tools to learn how well patients are adjusting. You will be given a tool to measure a patient's phase of adjustment and another to measure what coping skills are lacking.

PHASE OF ADJUSTMENT TO DISEASE

Patients move through phases in their adjustment. The following questionnaire describes reactions in five different phases. The first phase (items 1–10) is a *period of crisis* where there is tumult, disorder, and chaos. The second phase (items 11–20) is a *period of stabilization* where there is not necessarily adjustment but patients feel more steady and less besieged. The third phase (items 21–30) is a *period of alienation* where patients feel estranged and distanced from their body. The fourth phase (items 31–40) is a *period of feeling consolidated* where patients feels closer to their body, are more reconciled to having a disease, and feel more secure over all. The fifth phase (items 41–50) is a *period of synthesis* where patients feel adjusted to the limitations imposed by the disease and are finding meaning in their life even though there are physical changes. For a fuller description of these phases, read the Coping Skills Book.

Bear in mind that patients do not move through these phases in a linear way; there is not always "onward and upward." They may move back and forth between consolidation and crisis, depending on the presence of new symptoms or changes in the prognosis. They may not ever enter an alienation phase. They may have a short crisis, stabilize, and then begin to synthesize elements of their old and new life. Some patients never feel in crisis, adjust quite readily, and move directly into the synthesize phase.

HAND-OUT 5.1: *Phases of Adjustment to Disease****

People pass through different phases with their disease. We want to know what phase you are in. Check-off which answers apply to you.

_____   1.   I am still in shock about having this disease.

_____ 2. I am very alarmed and anxious about how this disease will effect my life and how it is effecting people close to me.

_____ 3. I feel so insecure since this disease happened to me, because it threatens what I care about.

_____ 4. Everything seems in chaos now. My life does not seem stable any more.

_____ 5. I feel like the life I knew is falling apart.

_____ 6. This disease (or the treatment for it) has changed or stopped so many of my habits, hobbies, and other activities I used to do.

_____ 7. Since I got this disease I do not care about the goals I used to work to accomplish.

_____ 8. My head feels like it is spinning since I got the news about having this disease, since I started having symptoms, or since the disease seems like it will change my life so much.

_____ 9. I think I am at a turning point in my life.

_____ 10. Since I found out about this disease, or since I started having symptoms, everything that I cared about feels like it is crumbling before my very eyes and I cannot stop it.

_____ 11. I am not as upset about having this disease as I used to be. I have gotten over a lot of the shock.

_____ 12. My life does not feel like it is in chaos anymore.

_____ 13. I am better able to cope now about having this disease.

_____ 14. I have gotten used to my symptoms or the fact that I have this disease.

_____ 15. My life has returned to being steady and stable.

_____ 16. I have gotten used to the suffering this disease causes me.

_____ 17. The suffering this disease causes me does not bother me like it used to do.

_____ 18. I have returned to most if not all of my old habits, routines, and normal activities.

_____ 19. I am handling not knowing what will happen in my future or what will happen to my body much better.

_____ 20. I feel like I am putting things back together again.

_____ 21. I don't really like my body anymore since I started having these symptoms or was told I have this disease.

_____ 22. I feel so different from other people since I started having these symptoms or since I found out I have this disease.

_____ 23. I am so angry with myself because I cannot fulfill all or part of my role duties like I used to do, or because I cannot meet all or some of other's expectations for me.

_____ 24. I cannot stand all of the changes in my body or the changes that will occur in my body in the future.

_____ 25. I blame myself completely or partly for getting this disease.

_____ 26. I am upset with certain people in my life because they do not seem to understand what it is like having this disease.

_____ 27. I am upset with certain people in my life because they have not given me the help I need now that I have this disease. I feel let-down by them.

_____ 28. I feel so all-alone having this disease.

_____ 29. I do not feel the same closeness I used to have with certain people since I got this disease.

_____ 30. Since I got this disease I feel distant from God and/or religion.

_____ 31. I do not feel as guilty any more about not being able to fulfill my role duties or about not meeting other's expectations.

_____ 32. I feel closer to the people I care about in my life.

_____ 33. My body has changed, but I am starting to understand it better now, regarding its limitations, when it can and cannot do certain things, and what I need to do for it.

_____ 34. I am not down on my body nearly as much as I used to be because it cannot be a certain way or cannot do certain things.

_____ 35. I am finding ways to manage the physical problems this disease causes me.

_____ 36. I am not upset like I was with some of the significant people in my life since my body starting changing.

_____ 37. I feel closer to my body now and appreciate it more.

_____ 38. I have gotten involved or gotten closer to other people since I got this disease and that has been helpful.

_____ 39. I feel closer to God now and/or more involved in religion now.

_____ 40. I have gotten over many of my bad feelings about getting this disease.

_____ 41. My life seems meaningful now, or more meaningful than it used to be since I got this disease.

_____ 42. I have found some new activities that are meaningful to me.

_____ 43. I have been able to resume some or all of my old activities that used to give my life meaning.

_____ 44. I feel like my life is coming together again.

_____ 45. I have gotten used to having this disease and doing what is necessary to treat it.

_____ 46. I have gotten used to my body not being able to do what it used to do before the disease.

_____ 47. I have goals I care about that I pursue.

_____ 48. Certain things have ended for me or will end but I feel okay about that now.

_____ 49. When I cannot do certain things or look a certain way because of this disease I know how to cope with that now.

_____ 50. This disease is just one part of my life now and is no longer dominating my thinking or attention.

While there is no exact cut-off indicating problems at any one phase of adjustment, if there are at least six items checked for a phase then that reveals that particular patient is in that phase of adjustment. Patients can also have facets of two phases of adjustment. For instance, they can check several items from 31–50, and that would mean that they feel consolidated and is in the process of synthesizing a new life. Patients may also have several checks from 1–10 and 21–30. That would mean that they feel in crisis and alienated. Providers also need to carefully look at clusters of checked items. For example, there may be alienation from others but no alienation from one's body.

CLINICAL INTERVIEW

Once providers know the approximate phase of adjustment, they need to probe further. The previous questionnaire needs to be supplemented with a clinical interview where the provider can ask open-ended questions. Following are sample questions.***

Crisis Phase Questions

1. Do you feel like you are in a crisis in your life now?
2. What is it like for you being in crisis? How well do you adjust to being in a crisis?
3. Are you used to being in a crisis in general? Is the feeling of crisis new to you or something you have experienced at other times in your life?
4. If you have been in other crisis before, how did you cope at that time? What made a difference?
5. Are there times when you do not feel like you are in a state of crisis? What is going on at that time? How are others acting at that time? What are you doing or what are you thinking so you do not feel like you are in a crisis? To get this positive situation again, what will you have to do again? What will you have to do again, to get your family members to do what you want so you are not in crisis? What would you be saying to yourself that would be different from when you feel like you are in a crisis?

6. Let us pretend that you wake up tomorrow and a miracle has occurred and you do not feel like you are in a crisis anymore, but you still have your disease and you still have to be treated for it. What will be different? How can you make this miracle happen? What could keep you from making this miracle happen?

7. What can you do to make this miracle happen just a little, say 20%? How could you make 50% of the miracle happen?

8. Is your family or anyone close to you in crisis because of your health problem? If so, how has their crisis affected you? Is it hard for you to manage when those close to you are in crisis? How would they have to change before you can ease your feeling of crisis? Do you feel guilty for causing them to be in crisis?

9. Who in particular would need to cope better before you can ease your crisis?

10. Are you fearful you will not be able to reach certain goals in your life now because of your disease? Are you afraid you will have to give up or forego certain dreams you have for your life?

11. How are you coping with treatment for your disease? Have you adjusted to the needs of treatment? Have you adjusted to the changes treatment has caused for you?

12. You may be finding that some duties you are not able to complete at this time. What do you say to yourself when you cannot complete your responsibilities, or meet other's expectations for you?

13. You may find that you are limited from doing certain things now. How do you handle being limited? Is it hard for you and if so, how hard from zero to ten?

Notes on above questions:

Questions 3 & 4 want to know how much crisis is a part of a patient's life. Is he or she crisis prone? Does he or she have a pseudo-crisis, when they do not have a real crisis but feel like they are in one? Questions 5–7 are from solutions oriented therapy (deShazer, 1985). Question 5 inquires about exceptions when the patient is not in crisis. Question 6 is the "miracle question," which fixes the desired outcome state where the patient sets a realistic goal for what can be accomplished, given his or her current reality.

Questions for Post-Crisis Phase:

1. Do you think your life is getting back to normal now? If so, how did you manage to take whatever steps you took to turn things around? What were you telling yourself that allowed you to stop feeling like you are in crisis?

2. What would "normal" be like for you?

3. What did you do to get yourself ready for a stable life again? How did you change your thinking or behavior to be able to resume a stable life?

4. Now that you have developed a stable life again and moved out of crisis, what does this say about you? What new picture do you have of yourself now that you have re-stabilized your life?

5. Did you like your normal life before you became sick?

6. Do you see any problems that could arise if your life goes back to normal and you resume your old routines?

7. Could going back to normal cause you to end treatment or not follow the doctor's recommendations?

8. Do you like having things feel stable or in some way do you enjoy a state of crisis? Is there anything attractive about a time of crisis to you? Do you like a calm, orderly existence or do you find it boring and too uneventful?

9. In the past, when things settled down after a crisis, did you stop doing what you needed to do to avoid crisis again?

10. Have you been on a medical regimen in the past or been in recovery from some type of addiction? If so, did you follow your program or vary it or drop it after a while?

11. Are you the kind of person who is compliant with the medical regimen? Have you ever been described as headstrong or too independent?

Notes on post-crisis questions:

Questions 1–5 are from narrative therapy (White & Epston, 1990). They invite patients to think about what they did to bring about change. Questions 5–8 inquire if the patient prefers a coping strategy that includes crisis as a way of living. Questions 9–11 inquire about what could de-stabilize the patient.

Questions for Alienation Phase

1. How do you like the person you have become since you got sick? Do you want to get rid of this new form of you? How much do you care about this new form of you? How much do you like or dislike yourself now that you have become sick?

2. How much has the disease taken over who you are as a person? How much of your basic essence (who you are as a person) has changed since you got this disease or started treatment?

3. Do you feel close to the person you are now or do you feel distant from who you are now?

4. Have there been changes in your relationships with others since you became sick? Are you closer or more distant to the significant people in your life now? Have you pulled away from others or have they pulled away from you?

5. If you are more distant from others, what is it like for you?

6. Are you a religious person in general? If so, has your participation in religious activities changed since you became sick? Do you still believe in God as much as you did before you became sick? Are you closer or do you feel more distant from religion and God since you became sick? Do you feel God has let you down? Do you think God has brought you this disease for some reason? Do you feel punished for something you have done? Do you blame God, fate, or fortune for your illness?

7. Things have gotten bad for you since your disease began. How come things are not worse? What are you doing to keep things from getting worse?

8. If you continue to feel alienated from your body (or from significant others in your life), what do you think will happen if things do not get better?

9. If that bad thing you just mentioned does happen, what will happen next, and then after that? What could make the smallest change to prevent those bad things from happening?

Notes on alienation phase questions:

Questions 1–3 ask about alienation from oneself. Questions 4 & 5 ask about alienation from others and question 6 asks about alienation from God. Question 7 is termed a coping sequence question (Berg & Gallagher, 1991). It is used for pessimistic patients who need to realize that things could be worse and that they are coping, but do not realize it. Questions 8 & 9 are pessimistic sequence questions (Berg & Gallagher, 1991) to raise anxiety to be more motivated to break out of the negative cycle of alienation—rejection of others or self—depression or anger—further alienation.

Questions for Consolidation and Synthesis Phases

1. What is it like for you when you encounter a limitation in yourself? What do you say to yourself not to be overwhelmed by a limitation? When you cope with limitations, how are you thinking and acting?
2. If you have had to give up some or all of your old activities, how much do you think about them?
3. What will you need to do to find peace-of-mind in your new life (or in the life you still have left)?
4. How confident are you on a scale from zero to ten that you can find a meaningful life now as a medical patient? What would you have to do to make that meaningful life happen?
5. How much do you think you have changed, from 0 to 10 with 10 being total change, since you first became sick? How did you manage to make that change?
6. If you were to gaze into a crystal ball regarding your progress since you became sick, what would you see about your future six months from now, or a year from now? What kind of changes would we see in that crystal ball?
7. If we were to make a videotape of you after you learned the different coping skills to manage these negative feelings you have to contend with, what would be on that videotape? How would you and others be acting and doing with one another?

Question 4 is a scaling question from solutions oriented therapy (de Shazer, 1985, 1991) to measure confidence about resolving the prevailing problems. Question 5 is a percentage question to measure change in the patient, also from solution-oriented therapy. Questions 6 & 7 are called future-oriented questions (Tomm & White, 1987) to increase positive anticipation about the future.

ASSESSING COPING SKILL DEFICIENCIES

Adjustment has a great deal to do with ability to cope. Inability to cope indicates a deficiency in one or more coping abilities. This section seeks to determine if there are coping skill deficits. The following questionnaire measures the deficits. The questions focus on several different emotions. The intent is to discover how well patients are able to tolerate and accommodate their emotions.

HAND-OUT 5.2: Your Response to Illness***

Below is a questionnaire that will help us learn what feelings you are having in your life now, what are problem feelings for you, and how much you feel those emotions. In answering the questions below, use the following answers:

0 = none at all
1 or 2 = hardly any at all
3 or 4 = a mild amount
5 or 6 = a moderate amount
7 or 8 = a large or extensive amount
9 or 10 = an exceptional amount

_____ 1. How much anxiety do you have most of the time?
_____ 2. How anxious are you about your future?

_____ 3. How well are you able to tolerate anxiety?
_____ 4. Since you became sick, how upset are you about not fulfilling your various duties?
_____ 5. Since you became sick, how much does it bother you when you do not meet other's expectations?
_____ 6. Do you feel much guilt now in your life?
_____ 7. Before you became sick, how much of the time did you find yourself feeling guilty?
_____ 8. When you cannot do what you want how much does that bother you?
_____ 9. How much frustration do you have in your life now?
_____ 10. How much have you grown accustomed to the frustrations that come with your illness?
_____ 11. How important is it to you to know what will lie ahead in your future?
_____ 12. How much would you say you are an easy-going kind of person, someone who can easily "go with the flow"?
_____ 13. Before you became sick, how optimistic of a person were you in general?
_____ 14. Now that you are sick, how optimistic are you about your future?
_____ 15. How much do you think about your future?
_____ 16. How much does uncertainty about what will happen to your body upset you?
_____ 17. How well are you living with uncertainty about the course of your illness?
_____ 18. How well are you able to cope with physical discomfort?
_____ 19. How well have you grown used to suffering since you became sick?
_____ 20. How much do you resent having to suffer because of your illness?
_____ 21. How much resentment do you feel most of the time?
_____ 22. How critical of your body are you?
_____ 23. How much do you feel that your body has let you down?
_____ 24. How much do you keep your anger inside?
_____ 25. How able are you to manage your anger?
_____ 26. How often do you feel disappointed in other people you care about?
_____ 27. How much do you feel disappointed in yourself since you became sick?
_____ 28. When your body cannot do something you want it to do, how disappointed do you get?
_____ 29. How down do you get when you are disappointed?
_____ 30. How well are you able to cope with disappointment?
_____ 31. How much do you think about what has disappointed you?
_____ 32. How upset do you get when you are deprived of what you want?
_____ 33. How much do you think about being deprived of what you care about?
_____ 34. How accustomed have you gotten to being deprived of what you care about because of your illness?
_____ 35. How much have you been rejected by others since you have become sick?
_____ 36. How much does rejection bother you in general?
_____ 37. How important is it to you to receive approval from people you care about?
_____ 38. How sad or down do you get when you are rejected?
_____ 39. If someone disapproves of you, how much do you think about that?
_____ 40. How important is it to you to be liked by others?

The questions deal with the following emotions:

Anxiety: questions 1–3

Guilt: questions 4–7

Frustration: questions 8–10

Uncertainty: questions 11–17

Suffering: questions 18–20

Resentment and anger: questions 21–25

Disappointment: questions 26–31

Deprivation: questions 32–34

Rejection and disapproval: 35–40.

In working with patients, providers need to be skilled in identifying the above feelings, regarding which is a problem for that patient. That will help providers form the treatment plan, by knowing which skills need to be taught and how much time needs to be given for training. On the disc is a skill building exercise ("Coping Skill Identification") for providers to help them develop skill in identifying appropriate skills for different situations medical patients face. Fill in the blanks and then check your answers against the author's answers.

GLOBAL ADJUSTMENT TO DISEASE

One way to measure adjustment is by learning how much a patient feels satisfied with his or her existence, given the perceived affects of the disease. What is being measured, then, is the "*subjective interruptive capacity" of a disease*: how much a patient believes her disease prevents her from gaining pleasure and finding meaning in her existence. In essence, we want to know how much harm a disease causes, and how much it interferes with finding a satisfying life, from the perspective of the patient. This will require two measurements: a subjective rating of life changes and an overall satisfaction score.

HANDOUT 5.3: How Much Has Your Disease Changed Your Life***

To answer that question, consider the following questions:

- How much has your disease impeded or prevented you from doing what you want to do?
- How much has it harmed your relationships?
- How much has it intervened in your activities, impeding your ability to pursue them?
- How much has it changed your basic roles and your ability to fulfill your role duties in the various parts of your life?

Now give your answer from 0 to 100, using the following guidelines:

0 to 25 = mild life effects; very little impact on goal attainment, relationships, role maintenance, and activity pursuits.

25 to 50 = moderate life affects; role maintenance and goal attainment have been disrupted but you can still sustain the lifestyle you had prior to your disease; your relationships are suffering to some extent but are still intact and stable.

50 to 75 = moderate to severe life affects; role maintenance has been altered in major ways; activity pursuits have been impeded significantly but can still be pursued; goals are attained much less of the time; relationships are either significantly damaged or are becoming unstable.

75 to 100 = severe to extensive life affects; old roles, activities, and meaningful pursuits have either been terminated or have changed significantly; goal attainment minimal; you believe barriers to goal attainment are insurmountable; your relationships have been terminated or have changed dramatically.

Now give your score: _____

We can call this measure the Subjective Disease Affects Score (SDAS). The SDAS score does not necessarily mean patients are upset about their life. A high score does not automatically lead to low life satisfaction. A disease can cause substantial suffering, but if the patient has proper coping skills then suffering can be managed. Consequently, in order to know how disease affects and life affects have influenced patient satisfaction, a second measure needs to be taken—the Life Satisfaction Score (LSS). This score shows overall life satisfaction.

*HANDOUT 5.4: What Is Your Satisfaction With Your Life?*****

To answer this question, use the following guidelines:

   0 to 25 = very low to abysmal life satisfaction.

   25 to 50 = low to moderate life satisfaction.

   50 to 75 = moderate to high life satisfaction.

   75 to 100 = high life satisfaction.

   Your Life Satisfaction Score: _____

To learn how well a medical patient copes in general, though, we also need an objective measure of actual anatomical damage and physical alterations resulting from disease. We can call this score the Objective Disease Affect Score (ODAS). The ODAS score is gleaned from a physical examination, testing, and laboratory results. Medical personnel will have to supply the ODAS. They can provide a global score of disease affects. The following continuum can be used for this purpose:

   0 to 25 = minor tissue or structural change

   25 to 50 = modest tissue or structural change

   50 to 75 = modest to severe tissue or structural change

   75 to 100 = severe to extensive tissue or structural change.

Usually in the early phase of a disease, an inverse relationship exists between life satisfaction and disease affects. A high score on the SDAS and the ODAS would lead to a low LSS. The reason is that in the early phase of a disease, coping skills have not had an opportunity to be developed, so when there is a major disruption in roles, activities, and relationships, and difficulty attaining pre-morbid goals, then that would cause low life satisfaction. However, as patients learn how to cope they are not as bothered as much by their disease and major life changes. When they move into the consolidation and synthesis phases, there should be a higher LSS score. At that time the disease can cause significant physical damage but there is greater capacity to cope with life problems.

If a medical patient in general has a high score on life satisfaction then that would indicate good adjustment and acceptance of changes forced on him or her. High scores on ODAS, SDAS, and LSS would indicate that a patient has not disallowed and rejected his or her disease, even though there are many negative changes in the body, role maintenance suffers, and goal attainment is lagging. Likewise, if a significant relationship has been terminated or dramatically altered, and the patient still has a high life satisfaction score, that would mean he or she has adjusted to his or her situation.

SUMMARY

Assessment tools are provided in this chapter to measure a patient's phase of adjustment. Five phases are described: crisis phase, stabilization phase, alienation phase, consolidation phase, and synthesis phase. To measure each phase, a questionnaire and clinical interview are provided. A second assessment tool is a questionnaire to measure coping skill capacity. Finally, providers are given a way to score a patient's global adjustment by considering his or her estimate of life satisfaction and perceived affects of disease.

Treating the Response to Suffering

Disease would not be a problem if someone did not have to suffer as a result of it. Suffering is a global negative feeling that includes such broad feelings as distress and misery. Its presence indicates something is not wanted and is disliked. It is composed of a combination of emotions like anger, frustration, or disappointment, physical sensations such as pain, throbbing, burning, or physical conditions such as weakness or fatigue. This chapter discusses how to assess suffering and how to come to terms with it as a quintessential aspect of the disease experience.

ASSESSMENT OF SUFFERING

Several factors can cause someone to suffer. Certainly one cause is a dysfunctional body that has unpleasant physical sensations or mechanical problems. Physical threshold for pain and emotional tolerance for distress also influences how much someone suffers. Another major cause of suffering is loss or harm to role functioning as a consequence of physical problems. Past suffering will influence how well someone can tolerate present suffering. Being at a disadvantage due to a disease also causes suffering, especially when the person does not permit being disadvantaged. As the disease continues people are forced to endure on-going pain, injury, and difficulty, and at some point they are not able to absorb further distress. There is little ability left to tolerate any more hurt, hassle, grief, trouble, or unpleasantness. This is *a secondary cause of suffering: distress due to suffering too much.* Yet, "too much suffering" is subjective and varies with the individual. Finally, suffering is due to an evaluation of one's situation. If someone characterizes his situation as terrible or awful then that will cause him to suffer even more.

In summary, providers need to assess several factors when they learn about a patient's level of suffering. The following three assessment tools (handouts 6.1, 6.2, 6.3) will give you information on the subjective disease experience, activating events stimulating that response, and the patient's response to suffering.

HANDOUT 6.1: Your Disease Experience***

We want to know how your disease has affected you. Please answer the following questions.

1. What is it like for you having this physical problem?
   a. Describe how you feel physically.
   b. Describe how you feel emotionally as a result of this condition.
   c. Describe how this condition has effected your relationships with others close to you.
   d. Describe how this condition has effected your work and job performance. What is your employer's response to your health problem?
   e. Over all, as a result of having this condition, how much distress are you feeling from 0 to 10, with 10 the absolute amount of distress you can experience? _____

---

2. How much distress did you have in your life before the disease developed? How did you cope with that distress? To answer that question, think about past times when you were in pain, felt distressed or endured losses or harm of any kind.

3. How much suffering do you think you will have to endure in the future as a consequence of having this disease? Do you think things will get worse? How much worse from 0 to 10, with 10 being absolutely the worst possible? _____

4. Has there been a point where you simply could not bear any more suffering in your life? What caused you to reach that point?

5. How would your loved ones describe your ability to cope when you are sick, from 0 to 10, with 10 being total ability to tolerate suffering? _____

HANDOUT 6.2: *What Causes You to Suffer?****

Check-off any of the factors below that cause you to suffer and how much misery you are experiencing as a result from 0 to 10. Use the following guideline when answering:

0, 1: little to no suffering

2, 3: suffering a mild amount

4, 5, 6: suffering a moderate amount

7, 8: suffering a severe amount

9, 10: extreme misery, suffering greatly.

_____ 1. Unpleasant physical sensations
       _____ a. physical pain
       _____ b. achy
       _____ c. throbbing
       _____ d. tingling
       _____ e. burning
       _____ f. bloating
       _____ g. itching
       _____ h. other negative sensations _____
_____ 2. Muscle weakness, unsteadiness
_____ 3. Loss of mobility and ability to get around easily
_____ 4. Fatigue, tiredness
_____ 5. Tremor
_____ 6. Stiffness, rigidity
_____ 7. Lack of sleep or problems sleeping
_____ 8. Problems in treatment
       _____ a. involved or complicated treatment
       _____ b. treatment is painful
       _____ c. treatment has too many side-effects
       _____ d. treatment interferes with other important life activities
       _____ e. treatment causes losses or problems in other areas of my life, such as work, marriage, sex life, etc.
       _____ f. dealings with doctors, nurses, or therapists are distressing (e.g., waiting time to see them, difficult personality of a provider)
       _____ g. dealings with insurance companies and HMOs
_____ 9. Too much uncertainty in my life caused by disease or treatment
_____ 10. Financial losses and financial uncertainty due to disease
_____ 11. Inability to perform normal role duties

_____ a. at home
_____ b. at work
_____ c. in hobbies
_____ 12. Inability to meet others' expectations:
_____ a. Expectations of spouse
_____ b. Expectations of children
_____ c. Expectations of parents
_____ d. Expectations of friends
_____ e. Expectations of employer
_____ f. Expectations of co-workers
_____ 13. Disrespect from others because of inability to perform normal role duties or meet others' expectations
_____ 14. Appearance changes due to disease or treatment
(specify: _____)
_____ 15. Surgical effects (e.g., loss of body tissue or parts of body due to surgery
(specify: _____)
_____ 16. Relationship changes due to disease
_____ a. relationship changes with spouse
_____ b. relationship changes with children
_____ c. relationship changes with friends
_____ d. relationship changes with employer or co-workers
_____ 17. Others are suffering due to my disease
_____ 18. Loss of old lifestyle
_____ 19. Too many hassles just to perform normal daily activities
_____ 20. Changes or fluctuations in my emotions due to disease or treatment
_____ 21. Loss of:
_____ a. employment (if applicable)
_____ b. marriage (if applicable)
_____ c. friendships (if applicable)
_____ 22. Overall rating of how much my disease has caused:
a.   my family to suffer _____
How much this bothers me? _____
b.   my friends to suffer _____
How much this bothers me? _____
c.   my employer to suffer _____
How much this bothers me? _____
d.   my co-workers to suffer _____
How much this bothers me? _____
_____ 22. Overall rating of my suffering _____ (from 0 to 100)

HANDOUT 6.3: _My Response to Suffering_***

The following is a check-list to learn how you may be feeling at this time in your life and how you may be responding to your disease and suffering. Check-off if you feel, think, or do any of the following:

_____ 1.   I frequently feel impatient and irritable.
_____ 2.   I frequently feel dejected, sad, or depressed.
_____ 3.   I feel overwhelmed by the number of hassles and frustrations in my life.
_____ 4.   I have a tendency to slip into self-pity and feel sorry for myself.
_____ 5.   I blame others, God, fate, or fortune for why I became sick.

_____ 6. I hate the symptoms of my disease.
_____ 7. I think that I cannot go on any longer feeling like I do.
_____ 8. I cannot accept my body as it is presently.
_____ 9. I think that life or God has not been fair to me.
_____ 10. I frequently think about the "good old days" before I became sick.
_____ 11. I frequently imagine waking up and feeling well again.
_____ 12. I routinely think about a cure being found for my condition.
_____ 13. I frequently complain about my symptoms.
_____ 14. I often find myself sighing, grunting, or groaning.
_____ 15. I doggedly pursue a cure for my medical condition even though my doctors have said that it will not go away.
_____ 16. I avoid any situation that can worsen my condition.
_____ 17. I often protest why I am stuck with this disease, and why I became sick, saying statements like, "Why me?", or "I'm sick of these symptoms."
_____ 18. I have thoughts about suicide although I am not serious about killing myself.
_____ 19. I have thoughts about suicide and I think that on some occasion I will be capable of killing myself.
_____ 20. I have become more withdrawn and do not engage others in conversation as much as I used to do.
_____ 20. I hate my life.
_____ 21. I have a difficult time focusing on other more pleasant matters, and instead stay focused on my physical problems.
_____ 22. I cannot accept being sick. I reject how my life has gone.
_____ 23. I feel upset with myself when I cannot do things easily as I used to before I became sick.
_____ 24. I try not complaining about my health but I cannot stop talking about how bad I feel.
_____ 24. A lot of what I discuss with others concerns my health.
_____ 25. People would be surprised to know how upset I am inside about having this disease.

The purpose of the response to suffering questionnaire (handout 6.3) is to assess how upset a patient is and how well he or she has adjusted to being a medical patient. To arbitrarily set a cut-off, if a patient has checked-off 13 or more items, that would indicate substantial dislike of his or her life and probable maladjustment. This should encourage providers to explore if there is rejection of suffering.

In regard to the answers on the causes of suffering questionnaire (handout 6.2), inquire about the following:

a) What would be an "acceptable level of suffering" for the patient for any factor scored seven or more? An acceptable level of suffering is the level where the patient can tolerate that problem, where the problem is not overwhelming.

b) What would have to change before suffering could end? Would there have to be a total resolution of the problem? Is the patient seeking a magical answer?

In assessing a patient's response to suffering and disease, providers should not assume that any given factor has to result in suffering, even if it appears to be quite distressing. That is because one person may not be bothered by the same matter that deeply troubles another person, if the former knows how to cope with that problem. Also, providers need to examine their own responses to causes of suffering, to learn if their response mimics the patient's response. If therapists identify with the patient's plight they can give a message that the patient's response makes sense when it does not.

CHALLENGING THE SUFFERING RESPONSE

Once providers know what causes a patient to suffer, and the amount the patient does suffer, there is a need to question if that level is warranted. The coping skills perspective is that suffering can be minimized if patients embrace the skills necessary to adequately respond to the distressful activating event. To ready patients for skill development, raise the following questions:

- "Does the problem that troubles you have to cause you to suffer as much as you do?"
- "Why does X (e.g., fatigue, the distress of your family) cause you to feel as miserable as you do?"

The next set of questions emphasizes the power of the individual. This is especially important with patients who feel particularly helpless.

- "Are you doomed to feel miserable because of this disease or is there something you can do about it?"
- "What has to be in place inside of you to minimize your level of suffering?"

These questions elude to the coping capacity of the individual, or the lack of it. They create the idea that the level of suffering is commensurate with the ability to cope. Implied in this is the cognitive behavioral position, that the activating event (e.g., pain, inability to ambulate) does not directly and automatically result in a given level of suffering (the response does not come from the stimulus). Instead, there is a mediating property—the executive beliefs that promulgate the coping response—that strongly influences the end result.

REJECTION VERSUS ASSIMILATION OF SUFFERING

Hand-out 6.3 will give an indication if the patient is adjusting to having a disease, or is using the maladaptive coping strategy of rejection of suffering. If the latter is detected, discuss some of the signs of it with the patient and define what is the strategy. The disc contains a check-off form (Handout 10) to detect signs of rejection of suffering. Understanding the rejection of suffering strategy is crucial, because it is the most important cause of maladjustment to disease. It is composed of the following executive beliefs:

- Refuse to co-exist with the presence of disease.
- Protest and complain about health to show disdain for the disease. Maintain unfavorable disposition to health status. Permission is given to feel highly frustrated and thoroughly dislike one's condition.
- Refuse to adjust to suffering because that would show willingness to live with its presence.
- Be unwilling to bear negative emotions about disease and its consequence, and instead permit the expression of negative emotions freely.

Discuss with the patient the drawbacks to rejection of suffering. For one, it emphasizes dissatisfaction with what has happened, which keeps the disease and its symptoms in the foreground of the mind. Two, it increases other negative emotions such as bitterness, helplessness, and disappointment. Three, it de-emphasizes the learning of constructive coping skills that promotes adjustment. Four, it perpetuates hatred of the disease which means the body is also hated. Because the person is inseparable from the body the strategy indirectly lowers self-regard. Five, it leads to less tolerance of symptoms of the disease because the focus is on the impossible task of removing them from the body. When the symptoms continue to be felt there is more consternation. Finally, if pain is a dominant symptom, it causes patients to feel a higher level of pain due to the evaluation that it is "awful" (Melzack & Wall, 1965).

The opposite coping strategy is assimilation of suffering, which is the single most important element leading to adjustment to disease. Inform patients about the elements of that strategy. Below are the executive beliefs for that coping strategy:

- Allow the disease to exist because it is the reality that has to be adjusted to for that moment in time.
- Co-exist with the disease even though it is not wanted. It is now a part of me so it needs to become just another element of myself.
- Come to terms with what is and accept the disease as one facet of my life.
- Promote tolerance of unpleasant feelings, sensations, and bodily dysfunction caused by the disease.

- Forgive my body, myself, or others for causing the disease. Do not live with rancor because that will cause more problems.
- Seek resolution of anger as soon as possible so it does not add to physical problems.

(For a fuller discussion of these two coping responses, see Sharoff, 2004).

Discuss with patients the benefits to an assimilation of suffering strategy. One, it de-emphasizes the disease and stresses what is satisfying in the patient's life. It makes the disease just one of many defining features of the individual, so that the disease is not foreground on the mind. Two, by emphasizing acceptance, tolerance, and forgiveness, there is less bitterness about having a disease and greater ability to cope with it. Hatred of the disease and its symptoms decrease, which allows patients to live with their condition more peacefully. This is especially important for the symptom of pain. Pain is not experienced as sharply when the evaluation of it is more mild (Melzack & Wall, 1965).

CREATING THE GOAL STATE

Because CCT is influenced by the principles of existentialism; the emphasis on choice and freedom to choose is critical (May, 1950). Medical patients are now at a crossroads in their treatment. They can decide on what the goal state will be and the strategy for managing their suffering. To induct patients into practicing assimilation of suffering instead of rejecting suffering, a handout is provided on the disc (handout 12) that discusses the benefits of the former and the drawbacks of the latter.

Below is a format that providers can follow when presenting the topic of assimilation of suffering.

1. Identify the activating events that precipitate suffering—the reality to which the patient has to adjust.
2. Identify the patient's response to the chronic or terminal illness.
3. Validate how the disease has harmed the patient. ("You had all these hopes for your future and now you face uncertainty."). Acknowledge his or her subjective state and if necessary concede that the patient does face an awful situation.
4. Educate the patient about common responses among other medical patients (e.g., "When people face a troublesome, burdensome situation, there is a temptation to reject reality because it looks so unpleasant"). This shows the universality of experiences.
5. Clearly identify the patient's coping strategy for his or her disease and suffering. Identify that person's particular signs that indicate rejection of suffering.
6. Checkout if the patient agrees that he or she practices that coping strategy.
7. Discuss what coping skills can lessen the level of suffering.
8. Inquire if the patient is willing to learn those skills.

If the patient chooses to practice the assimilation of suffering strategy, there are many techniques that can facilitate it. Sharoff (2004) has listed seven tactics for that purpose: a) self-instruction training, b) imagery (Sheikh, 1983) c) therapeutic metaphors (Gordon, 1978) d) symbolic gesturing, e) outcome enactment, f) enacting the role model, and g) anchoring (King, Novik, & Citrenbaum, 1983).

TREATING RESISTANCE

There will be patients, though, who hesitate or refuse to embrace the assimilation of suffering response. This section presents several tactics and techniques that can be used to treat resistance.

1.   Illuminating the Full Position

When patients reject further suffering, it is because they believe that their illness results in too much distress. From the standpoint of cognitive restructuring (CR), patients need to realize that a major reason for why they suffer is because of how they think. Likewise, resistance to assimilation of suffering is because of how patients think. Hence, changing patient thinking decreases resistance (Ellis, 1985).

One way to change patient thinking is by presenting a patient's full position on a matter. Part of the position is often in the subconscious and is not known to the patient. The part that is consciously known seems reasonable to the person only because the full position has not been explicated and clarified. Bringing out the "full position" on a subject often reveals irrationality or unrealistic thinking. The patient is then asked if she still subscribes to that point of view.

To increase your ability to explicate someone's full position, two common responses among medical patients are reported. The therapist then reports the patient's full position on that subject, which is often not consciously known.

Belief A#

Patient: "It's not right how my life has gone, to become sick and feeble."

Therapist: "Are you saying, 'I should only be well, that that is the only right thing that can happen to me, that I am meant to be healthy, and only being healthy should happen to me?' "

Belief B#

Patient: "I am so angry with my HMO for giving me such a hard time."

Therapist: "What I am hearing you say is, 'My HMO should not manage my care, not limit my treatment, and not try to save itself money. My HMO should pay for whatever I need, which would be best for me, but at a cost to the HMO. My HMO should not think about money and put patients first. In other words, my HMO should not operate like an HMO, or at least be a benign, enlightened HMO operating in the way I think best.' "Upon hearing the full position with its irrational ideation, many patients automatically surrender their thinking. Disputation is often not needed at this point.

2. Forced Choice Technique

This cognitive restructuring technique (Wessler & Wessler, 1980; McMullin, 1986) asks patients to take an objective stance and hear two responses to suffering side-by-side—one irrational and the other rational. They are then asked to select which one causes the most problems and which will yield the least negative emotion. First, patients hear the rejection of suffering response: "I hate this disease. It stinks. I am miserable and it is all the fault of this damn body that cannot heal up." Then, the mind-set of assimilation of suffering is presented: "I do not like what is happening to me but I cannot change reality. It is not wanted but I have to deal with it. I can work to bear what is happening to me. I don't want to live my life hating my situation and crying over spilled milk." Obviously the latter will yield the least negative feeling, pressuring the patient to adopt this mind-set.

3. Self-Instruction Training

Self-instruction training (Meichenbaum, 1977; Meichenbaum & Jaremko, 1983) is helpful for developing the capacity to assimilate suffering and stress into one's life. It also has benefit for overcoming rejection of suffering (hand-out 6.4 below).***

HANDOUT 6.4: Overcoming Rejection of Suffering

Preparing for situations where I may reject further suffering:

Has my suffering increased in situations like this in the past?
Have I fallen into rejecting suffering in similar situations?
If I have, be ready to deal with that way of coping. It is not helpful.

Do not get into demanding to be someone physically who I cannot be right now.
Do not get into believing my future is bleak. Take one day at a time.
Hating this disease makes me hate my life. Give-up the hate. It provides no benefit.
I do not have to like having a disease but I do have to accept that I have one.
Live with reality. Stop the protest against it. Adjust to what is.
Don't fall into brooding. Side-step self-pity. That only causes dejection.
Monitor signs of rejection of suffering.

Dealing with a situation when rejection of suffering is noticed:

I am feeling worse now. I notice that I am rejecting suffering in this situation.
Do not get mad about suffering. Do not get discouraged and dejected. That will only make me
    feel worse.
Bear up to an increase in suffering.
I cannot drive out suffering. It is a part of me now that I have this disease.
Do not disallow it. Stop the protest against it. Stop focusing on it.
I do not want to suffer but it cannot be avoided. Live with it. Let it into my life. It is a part of
    my existence.
I suffer enough. Do not increase my suffering by hating how my life is.

Dealing with oneself after the situation has ended:

Monitor for signs of dejection or anger about discomfort in this situation. How much distress am
    I carrying with me right now?
Refocus on other matters that are pleasant. Don't stay focused on the problems in my body.
Take a few deep breaths and relax. Let go of the physical tension from suffering.
Do not hate my life because it is not as healthy as it used to be.
Do not carry around resentment about how my life is now. Adjust to what I have to face. Do not
    get into wishful thinking. Accept who I am.

In addition to the above self-dialogue, the disc contains two self-dialogues to help patients cope with suffering. One covers managing suffering while engaged in activities (handout 14) and the second addresses acceptance of self when engaging in work (handout 15). That dialogue specifically targets anger about not being one's "good ol' self."

4. Prescribed Coping Rituals

An adaptation of the Milan family therapy technique (Boscolo, Hoffman, & Penn, 1987) can be used to show patients how ill-advised rejection of suffering actually is. First, therapists list the mind-set and actions of both rejection of suffering and assimilation of suffering. Next, patients are asked to practice rejection of suffering on odd days of the week, and assimilation of suffering on even days of the week. This lines up each response set side-by-side and a patient then selects the strategy that causes the most problems and the one that helps the most.

5. Incentive Analysis

CCT uses an incentive analysis (Edwards, 1954) to help patients dispassionately assess the viability and utility, the pros and cons, of rejection of suffering. Next, the pros and cons of assimilation of suffering are listed. Finally, the patient selects which response has the most benefit.

This technique is used because patients are loyal to maladaptive strategies but are often unaware of why. The technique brings the so-called benefits to the surface (e.g., opportunity to gain revenge against another person). Once aware of the incentives to sustain a maladaptive strategy, people can then intellectually weigh if that is the best course to take in comparison to other tactics.

6. Relapse Prediction

Providers should tell patients to be prepared to face resistance to assimilation of suffering. Patients should be warned that they will probably relapse at various times and resume protesting, self-pity, self-hatred, and self-criticism for becoming ill or not healing, and they need to be ready when that happens. That is because frustration about having a disease is strong and the penalties from being ill are widespread. Because of that there will be difficulty sustaining assimilation of suffering. This is due to the human tendency to reject what is negative and not allow it into one's life. Knowing relapse will occur prepares patients to make use of techniques (e.g., self-instruction training) learned in treatment to override resistance to assimilation of suffering.

This tactic is especially recommended for patients who suddenly and easily make the switch to assimilation of suffering. Therapists need to worry that these patients have not worked through negative emotions about disease and instead will relapse back to rejection of suffering upon leaving treatment. This tactic is done to place patients in a therapeutic double bind. If they do not relapse, then that means that they are practicing assimilation of suffering, which places distress under the patients' control and that is desirable. If they do relapse and reject further suffering, then that means that they are neglecting to use the techniques learned in therapy. Warning them in advance that this will happen puts the deteriorating condition under the patient's control, and that is desirable (Seltzer, 1986; Weeks & L'Abate, 1982, 1985).

7. Scheduled, Limited, Planned Relapses

Patients who are ambivalent about surrendering their strategy of rejection of suffering can be given a recommendation to elect to reject suffering when they need to do so. In that case the relapse is planned. This paradoxical strategy (Seltzer, 1986; Zeig, 1980) places the patient in a double bind. If the patient chooses to reject suffering and ends up feeling worse as a consequence, then this reveals that the increase in suffering is due to the patient practices and not the disease itself. If the patient shuns a relapse and instead elects to practice assimilation of suffering and feels better as a consequence, then this shows that he or she is able to avoid higher levels of suffering by choosing to practice this coping strategy.

In this technique, patients are told that when they feel unable to cope, they can purposely become irrational and plan a meltdown for a prescribed time period. This is a *scheduled breakdown* in rational functioning. During that time they give themselves permission to feel sorry for themselves and vent about their misfortune until the time period is up. At that time they must return to the mind-set of assimilation of suffering.

8. Forced Responsibility-Taking

While many patients realize the hazards and repercussions from rejection of suffering, they nevertheless revert back to that response because of their antagonism against and hatred of their disease. CCT addresses this problem by asking patients to take responsibility for their response. The negative consequences from rejection of suffering are listed and patients are asked to accept those consequences if they elect to pursue that strategy.

9. Contextual Search

This technique from CCT (Sharoff, 2002) recognizes the idea that every pathological response contains positive coping skills and seeks to make use of those skills where they are appropriate. Specifically, the rejection of suffering response is comprised of beneficial responses that need to be "contextualized" in the appropriate time and place, and when that occurs the response is no longer problematic.

For example, rejection of suffering contains an agonistic tendency to battle against forces harming oneself. That response is problematic when used in the context of blaming fate or fortune for causing distress. In that context it moves patients to fret and bemoan their plight. However, using a contextual search, appropriate contexts for an agonistic tendency are discovered, such as physical therapy where patients are asked to challenge their body to overcome physical limitations, or when battling against dying from a terminal condition. Another essential element of rejection of suffering is protest. When used in the context of family life it causes patients to endlessly complain about their symptoms, which only alienates loved ones from them. The positive contexts for using protest are then prescribed, such as when a physician is not offering adequate information and the patient protests the doctor's behavior.

10. *Restraining Technique*

This paradoxical tactic (Weeks & L'Abate, 1982; Seltzer, 1986) is used with ambivalent patients who inconsistently practice assimilation of suffering techniques, or who are slow in making progress. To address this resistance, they are discouraged from using assimilation of suffering techniques and instead are encouraged not to progress too fast or too soon. The reason given is that the patient may not be ready to feel better at that point in time. "You seem to have a higher need to express negative feelings about having your disease. While expressing those negative feelings will cause you to feel worse, it does appear to be a more pressing need than moving on with your life and make suffering a part of your existence. I suggest holding back on feeling better because that will address your immediate need to protest and hate your illness." This tactic indirectly encourages defiance against restraining change, and by defying the therapist the patient practices assimilation of suffering techniques which is what is desired.

11. *Prescribing Coping Skills for Maladaptive Responses*

This is a coping skills approach that has a paradoxical intention. Patients are told to maintain their maladaptive response but if they choose to do so then certain skills will become necessary in order to cope. Therapist: "You choose to reject suffering and disallow the existence of your disease. In that case you will need *pain management training*, because you will have more pain as a result. You will need *anger management* and *frustration tolerance*, because you will end-up more angry and frustrated. That is because rejection of suffering will increase your anger and frustration."

This tactic is advisable for chronic pain patients who are angry about having their injury. They are told to continue to stay that way if they choose but they will need to learn discomfort amelioration skills (Sharoff, 2004) in that case. That is because they will have a higher level of physical discomfort when they hate and reject their pain. Hatred of their condition will literally make patients up-tight and increase muscular tension and inflammation.

In this technique, patients benefit either way. If they comply with the prescription and learn the skills, then they learn responses that can help them if they do reject suffering. If they hear the therapist's idea that they are causing their own problems to some extent, then they may be willing to stop their maladaptive response to disease.

12. *Therapeutic Metaphors*

Another way to treat resistance is to appeal to the unconscious mind and work to change it indirectly through the use of therapeutic metaphors (Gordon, 1978; Gordon & Myers-Anderson, 1981). In this technique, therapeutic metaphors are presented to patients without their conscious knowledge that the therapist is trying to change their thinking.

In the following example, a metaphor is given to a chronic back pain patient suffering from discogenic disease. The therapist uses the metaphor to support the use of the skill of Gestalt management, which is the ability to replace a negative foreground image with a positive, enhancing image (Sharoff, 2004). However, the patient has resisted using this technique and instead continues to complain about his injury. To overcome rejection of suffering and to encourage the use of Gestalt management, the following metaphor is used. The metaphor is given as *part of chitchat* between the therapist and unsuspecting patient.

Therapist: "Not that long ago I drove a long way to see this garden that is famous for its beauty. The problem was that the day was extremely hot and the humidity was very high, so the heat felt overwhelming and unpleasant. Yet, in between my complaints and protest about the heat, I noticed that I was not even looking at the garden very intently. I was seeing it but not looking at it. I was not noticing the beauty of the place. I then tried to make the best of the day and paid close attention to the positive details in how the garden was laid out. I saw the matching and contrasting colors, the use of different flowers to make a certain look. When I started getting into the details of the scene, I noticed that I was unaware of the heat."

In this metaphor the therapist compares the patient's disease to a hot and humid day. The patient is compared to the therapist where both are acting similarly. A solution for suffering—Gestalt management—is also given metaphorically as looking at the colors in the garden (replacing a negative foreground image with a positive one) instead of focusing on what is causing suffering, the oppressive heat.

13.   Monitoring and Evaluation

Self-management techniques (Rokke & Rehm, 2001) can be used with patients who consciously agree that rejection of suffering is counter-productive but nevertheless slip back into that response mode, due to their antagonism toward their illness. Without realizing it, patients allow their resentment about their disease to be expressed as protest. One way to treat this problem is by utilizing self-monitoring and self-evaluation, which acts to increase conscious awareness of unconscious influence. Using handout 6.5, patients then monitor when they are non-compliant to the psychological regimen.

HANDOUT 6.5: Self-Evaluation Form to Detect Rejection of Suffering***

1.   What was the highest amount of distress that I felt today, from 0 to 5, with 5 being the most I could possibly suffer from having this condition (e.g., illness)?
2.   Did I fall into self-pity or bitterness about having this illness today? Yes _____ No _____ What were the signs of rejecting my suffering today? _____
3.   Did I accept the fact that I will suffer from having this illness? Yes _____ No _____ Did I hate my illness or make it a part of my life, a normal part of my existence? _____
4.   Did I endure my suffering from having this illness? Yes _____ No _____ Did I endure the losses, pain, and deprivation that comes from having this disease?
5.   Did I feel proud of myself for how well I withstood the unpleasantness from having my illness? Yes _____ No _____
6.   What techniques did I use to help me assimilate my suffering into my life, and if so, rate its effectiveness from 0 to 5, with 5 being extremely helpful?
     a)   Self-talk; rating _____
     b)   Imagery; rating _____
     c)   Symbolic gesturing; rating _____
     d)   Anchoring; rating _____
     e)   Anything else _____; rating _____

SUMMARY

This chapter provides three forms to assess suffering. One assesses the disease experience, another identifies situations that cause suffering, and the third identifies the response to disease. Providers are asked to challenge the idea that the disease causes suffering and instead look to the maladaptive coping response of rejection of suffering. The substitute coping response of assimilation of suffering is discussed, which promotes acceptance of the disease and tolerance of it. Numerous tactics are given to treat resistance to assimilation of suffering.

Identity and Self-Esteem Management

Identity is the recognition of self. From the multitude of traits, roles, and actions undertaken by a person, a self-definition emerges, and when that happens someone has a "This is me" moment that marks who the self is. Identity selects facets of the individual and equates the self to them.

From this process a feeling about the self is reflexively formed. If the feeling feels good, then the individual experiences self-esteem while approving of himself. Self-esteem is not only a sentiment about oneself but also cognition as well, a special type of value judgment that declares, "I am good and have worth."

With the advent of disease, though, a critical juncture occurs in identity processing. Identity is subverted by a stream of negative self-perceptions. Disease inevitably infiltrates, confiscates, and perverts identity while diminishing self-esteem. Too often, whatever positive self-regard existed is sullied by ill-health; self-esteem diminishes as the medical patient cannot look or perform like he or she previously did.

Managing the affect of disease on identity and self-esteem readily becomes a major treatment issue. Because disease affects cannot be avoided, patients must be converted into being an *active watchdog* to detect pernicious influences on self-concept and feelings about the self. This is the process of **identity management**, where the influence of situations and bodily dysfunction are mediated by an *internal inspector* that passes judgment on perceptions of self, declaring them acceptable or non-acceptable. The latter are then eliminated if deemed injurious or toxic to well being.

The inspector seeks to avoid three types of identity crisis:

1. **Identity adulteration** is the sullying of a positive self-image, producing a lowering of self-esteem. This results in a re-organization of foreground images about the self. Some images that used to dominate attention are pushed into the background and new images that are essentially negative in nature become foreground.
2. **Identity alienation** occurs when that adulterated image is too repugnant to be integrated into the definition of self. To protect self-image and to avoid a lowering of self-esteem, estrangement from self ensues. The individual dissociates from and feels unfriendly toward the new self affected by disease, seeing it as the Not-Me. The Old Me, the Essential Me, is preserved while the Not-Me is viewed with contempt. "That person there, hobbled by an aching back, walking like he has one foot in the grave, is not me. 'I' appear later in the morning when I start to feel better and stronger, when I emerge as my old self."
3. **Identity loss** occurs when desired positive self-percepts diminish and evaporate, leaving a meager and insufficient assemblage of traits and facets of self to form the foundation for identity. The new version of self cannot support a healthy self-concept. Favored features of identity are demoted or eliminated, and when this occurs a subtle erosion or dramatic plunging in self-esteem happens.

We will now turn our attention to how to avoid these three identity crises. Two skills for managing identity will be discussed: **identity scrutiny** and **identity coalescing**. Their use with one manifestation of identity—**identity markers**—is presented. Ways to support and develop self-esteem are given, including the activities of **self-boosting**, **self-compassion**, and **self-advocacy**. One problem area that lowers self-esteem receives particular attention, the issue of guilt.

IDENTITY COALESCING

Because disease and treatment cause significant changes in identity, medical patients need to engage in a task of coalescing their premorbid identity with the identity formed since disease onset. This task is called **identity coalescing**.

This task has several component tasks. One, if a facet of the old identity was positive, then patients need to preserve that facet as much as possible. This means maintaining the source of that identity as much as possible. The source can arise from a role, relationship, avocation, or ownership of something (e.g., home, car, etc.).

Two, the identity of medical patients also has to include or make room for percepts of self as a chronic or terminal illness patient. That is because one important goal of treatment is integration of disease, whereby it becomes an accepted part of oneself. That includes seeing oneself in a benign way even with the presence of disease.

Three, the coalescing of images needs to be broad, where many views of self is included in the mix of images. Identity should not be based on a few qualities. If it is, then the patient is engaging in reductionistic thinking and cognitive restructuring needs to address that problem.

Four, identity coalescing needs to overcome "premature identity formation." That is, identity will fluctuate, shift, and change as the disease progresses, goes into remission, or returns. Patients will not know the uncertain courses their disease can take. Any given course can affect identity. Yet, future identity will not be known by watching and conceptualizing oneself on a day-by-day basis. But many chronic and terminal illness patients prematurely define who they are or will become cross-sectionally. Instead, they need to think longitudinally and redefine themselves over and over again across time. To do this they must take a "wait and see" attitude before concluding, "This is who I am or will be."

Five, identity coalescing needs to be present centered and dynamic. This means managing the perceptual flow, so one or a few actions do not dominate attention and drive other aspects of identity into the background. If only a few aspects of identity receive notice fixed or frozen Gestalts structure self-concept. Instead, identity needs to have *fluid and ever-changing Gestalt formations.* For instance, Daryl, a MS patient, sees himself as a gimp because he walks in an awkward way due to his disease. He has a fixed Gestalt formation. Yet, when seated, he can have a totally different experience of himself as compared to when he is walking. When seated, Daryl does not require as much neuromuscular control over his legs as when he is walking. Spasticity is not as much of a problem for him at that time. When seated he can notice other aspects of current functioning. His identity can shift to other images of self (e.g., as a conversationalist, as a wit). Hence, by maintaining fluid Gestalts of self, Daryl's identity can vary depending on what he is doing and embrace other percepts when the activity changes.

There are several matters that need to be assessed to facilitate identity coalescing.

1) Assess the patient's present identity. Ask for descriptions of self, or how the patient would describe him/herself to others.
2) Inquire what led to the present identity. What made that person proud of himself in the past and present? What roles, interests, or pursuits were staples of identity?
3) Assess the patient's past identity. Ask for descriptions of the premorbid self.
4) How has past identity changed as a consequence of having a disease? What facets of the old identity are still in operation?
5) What were the key activities in that patient's life that, without their existence, the person would suffer severe identity loss? Has the patient lost those activities in the present, and if so, how has that affected him or her?
6) Which are the patient's beliefs about what parts of identity have been lost and are those beliefs accurate? Is the patient being realistic or unrealistic regarding lost identity?
7) How much does the new identity dominate self-concept and eclipse the premorbid identity? Draw a pie chart to assess what parts of identity are premorbid and what parts have developed since disease onset.
8) Assess how much the patient is rejecting aspects of his or her new identity.

IDENTITY MARKERS: LOST AND FOUND

Identity loss is a very subtle process. In part it occurs through a loss of what can be called an *identity marker.* They are something that substantiate a facet of self, and make it appear distinct and easy to recognize. They tell the self, "This is me" and "I am still the same way." They confirm who the self is, and give evidence about who the self is. They are detected by either the conscious or unconscious mind. There are countless identity markers and using or possessing them congeals self-recognition and reaffirms identity. For example:

- The performance of an activity (e.g., riding a motorcycle, chauffeuring children, doing crafts)
- Body parts (e.g., testicles, breasts, genitals, thin ankles, broad shoulders, barrel chest)
- Tools (e.g., computer, wood-working tools, stethoscope, lawnmower)
- Items of clothing (e.g., three-piece suit, items with a brand label on them)
- Possessions (e.g., furniture, house, car)
- Living in a particular neighborhood (e.g., the wrong side of the tracks, the rich part of town).

There are many identity markers concerning chronic illness, such as medication, the use of a cane or wheelchair that denote the identity of a disabled person, or sloping shoulders and sagging chin that mark the identity of chronic fatigue. Repeated facial grimaces and groans denote "I am a chronic pain patient."

When people encounter an identity marker, they are having an experience that affirms who the self is. Below are some examples:

- Beth, a middle aged woman, puts on a tight fitting skirt and looks at her profile in the mirror. She touches her flat stomach and holds it for a moment. It is her identity marker and it reaffirms her membership in the trim, attractive, youthful female group.
- Ralph was just criticized and put-down by his wife. He stands up, pulls up his pants under his massive, overhanging stomach, puffs out his chest and chin, and walks away indignantly. He has just had an identity marker experience where he reaffirmed his self-image as a strong, tough, and powerful male, to counteract the negative effect that his wife just had on his self-esteem.
- Bill puts on his three-piece suit, grabs his brief case, and walks out the door to get into his BMW. Each is an identity marker that he is a successful, upper middle class businessman.

In chronic and terminal illness, positive identity markers are lost and when that happens people lose some facet of their identity. At the same time, new identity markers emerge that are usually negative, such as a limp or yellowish skin. Those markers adulterate the old identity.

Example A

Beth had to take a drug that caused her to gain substantial weight. She lost her trim, youthful identity and instead saw herself as an overweight, unkempt, fat slob (identity adulteration).

Example B

Ralph got cancer and lost his massive girth that was a positive identity marker for him. While looking trim, his new identity was of a weak, puny person. He felt alien and alienated from his new physique. To him, his lean look was the identity of a cancer patient, a sick, diseased person. His overall identity is adulterated by changes brought about by the disease and the treatment for it.

Example C

Bill got multiple sclerosis and with that he incurred the loss of numerous identity markers. His clear, quick mind felt dizzy and confused on many occasions, forcing him to stop driving his BMW. Forced to go on disability, he no longer needed to wear his three-piece suits each day. Each of these identity markers had supported his image of intellectual and social worth.

THERAPEUTIC STRATEGIES

Below are several strategies using identity markers.

Strategy 1. Rekindle and preserve the old identity marker to minimize identity loss. Case example: Bill felt inadequate, like a has-been, when he was forced to leave his job due to medical reasons. He deeply missed his identity as a powerful man in charge, a "mover and a doer." The therapist asked, "When you were working, when did you like yourself the most? What activities were you doing when you felt good about yourself?" Bill responded that he felt good about himself when he held his powerful position of general manager, which conferred status and respect. The therapist inquired how Bill looked when he acted as a man in charge. While Bill was unsure his wife said he always seemed powerful to her when he held up his chin, pulled his head back, and talked in a firm, low, deep, voice. Concluding this was an identity marker, and to regain his former identity of a power player, the therapist encouraged Bill to assume this "power pose" and "power voice" when he talked to others, especially health providers. While Bill no longer held the position that made him feel powerful, he could still maintain his identity if he could recapture how he projected power. The identity marker was his link to that lost identity.

Strategy 2. Develop new identity markers to maintain the old identity and avoid identity loss. Case example: Beth gained weight and lost her identity marker of a flat stomach that supported her identity as a desirable and attractive woman. Her therapist worked to find other ways to maintain that old identity. At various times in their discussions, Beth would have a gleam in her eye, look coy, tilt her head, and have a playful laugh. The therapist asked Beth if she liked herself at that moment and she replied affirmatively. He suggested that she use that look and playful laugh purposefully when interacting with others, to give her a feeling of being desirable and attractive. That new identity marker became the link to her old identity that she wished to preserve.

Strategy 3. Emphasize other facets of the old identity that were not prominent and build an identity marker as a link to them. This makes other images of self foreground instead of being in the background. This is helpful when an image that supported self-esteem has been lost or diminished. Case example: The fatigue and weakness from Beth's illness has caused her to feel sluggish and drained and unable to initiate action easily. Her vigor used to be an important part of her old identity. Her therapist emphasized, though, that Beth showed determination by still going to work regularly. He asked if she thought of herself as a determined person in general. She replied that she knew she was that way but being that way was not a major part of her identity. To make that image of herself more prominent, the therapist worked to build an identity marker for that quality. He suggested that she develop a look of determination, and don that look when she wanted to press forward, even with a lack of energy. The determination look included a tightening of her chin, a squinting of her eyebrows, and a biting on her lower lip. In essence, the look would stimulate the determination response. In time it became a more dominant and less recessive part of her identity.

Strategy 4. Build new features of identity to overcome identity loss. Form an identity marker to support and enjoy the new facet of identity. Case study: Ralph experienced identity loss because of his cancer. His therapist commented that Ralph presents himself gracefully and with dignity, especially when he is sitting down. Ralph would drape one leg carefully over the other and straighten his backbone as he sat. The therapist asked Ralph if he thinks of himself as graceful and Ralph replied that is not part of his self-image. The therapist then asked Ralph if he would like to think of himself that way and Ralph replied affirmatively. The sitting position then became the identity marker to the self-image of gracefulness.

IMAGE SCRUTINY

Unwittingly, inevitably, we receive feedback about ourselves from others, and that feedback creates images of ourselves. Those images say, "This is who you are." Images can be given nonverbally, such as by looks, intonation of voice, or what others do or not do with us (e.g., not including a coworker for lunch). Images are created verbally, through statements and critical comments. We also relate to ourselves as an object and give images to ourselves about who we are. The passing on of images is a subtle process and in so many cases we are not aware that it is occurring. However, a positive or negative feeling tells us that a new image of ourself has been received.

Usually, though, people do not scrutinize the images that they receive, but medical patients need to do that regularly. Daily, they need to be engaged in *image scrutiny.* That is because they constantly receive many negative images of who they are and that can lower their self-esteem and adulterate their identity.

Image scrutiny will identify the new image and decide if it should be integrated into the other images of self. Image scrutiny has a *gatekeeper function*. It may reject the new image as inaccurate or accept it if accurate.

To develop medical patient's ability to examine incoming images, a worksheet can be given to patients to guide them through image scrutiny. Hand-out 7.1*** is given to patients to examine the validity of other's view of them. The disc contains a handout for patients to help them scrutinize their images of themselves (handout 18). The handouts have three purposes: a) to increase self-awareness of images foisted on oneself (by others or oneself), b) to collect data to assess the validity of an image, and c) to collect data to dispute thinking about that image. In essence, image scrutiny leads into cognitive restructuring with oneself.

HANDOUT 7.1: *Scrutinizing Others' Views of Self*

1. After I interacted with _____, how did I feel, from −10 to +10, with +10 being feeling great about myself, or −10 being feeling terrible about myself?

2. In my interaction with _____, how did he/she relate to me? How did he/she see me or think of me?

3. How would I know that was _____'s image of me? What am I basing my thinking on? What is my evidence that _____ actually thinks of me that way?

4. Did I do anything to make _____ think of me that way?

5. If there is not enough data to conclude _____ thinks of me that way, should I discard the idea that _____ thinks of me that way? Yes _____   No _____

6. If I think there is reason to conclude _____ thinks of me a certain way, do I think of myself that way as well? Am I in agreement that I am this way as well? Yes _____   No _____

7. Do I think this way of thinking of myself is correct? Am I actually this way? Is this a valid view of myself?

8. If I think of myself as that way, how does that influence my view of myself, as good or bad. Rate how good or bad I think of myself from −10 to +10, with −10 being thinking of myself as the worst and +10 thinking of myself as the best. If my answer is −6 to −10 to question 8, answer the following questions: What makes it awful to be this way? Is it really awful to be this way or just not preferable to be this way? What are the benefits in being this way? Do I gain anything by being this way?

To know when to initiate the use of the previous worksheets, patients need to be encouraged to *self-monitor* their emotions. The presence of a negative or positive feeling indicates that an image has been received and needs to be scrutinized.

BUILDING SELF-ESTEEM

Functioning in one's roles may or may not increase self-esteem. However, dysfunction in a role will decrease self-esteem, maybe not immediately but over time esteem will erode when expectations for oneself continue to not be met. This is a major problem for medical patients, because their disease routinely interferes with role performance and activities of daily living. Likewise, the sense of self as disfigured will produce a loss of self-esteem.

Hence, one of the major tasks of medical patients is refurbishing, maintaining, or building damaged self-esteem. To accomplish this an on-going self-support capacity can be developed. Three self-support activities are emphasized for medical patients (see Coping Skills Book for fuller discussion of them):

1) ***Self-boosting:*** to habitually stress positive qualities and actions while de-emphasizing negative qualities and actions. In part, this is a perceptual ability to notice some aspects of performance while giving less attention to other aspects of self.

2) ***Self-compassion:*** to seek a nurturing way of relating to oneself. In part this involves giving permission not to act in expected ways or excusing oneself from meeting a standard. It involves a show of mercy to oneself when poor role performance occurs.

3) ***Self-advocacy:*** to defend oneself as needed when others or oneself are critical of role performance. This also involves justifying non-performance, protecting one's interests, and educating others about the patient's needs.

To develop these abilities, a self-management strategy is used (Rehm & Rokke, 1988; Rokke & Rehm, 2001). The above components of self-support are first discussed with the patient. She or he is asked to self-monitor if those components are being pursued daily. A check-off form (handout 7.2) is used in this effort. Finally, the patient evaluates the effectiveness of self-support in raising self-esteem.

HANDOUT 7.2: *Developing Self-Support****

Below are three activities that show support for yourself. Are you doing those activities daily? Check-off all that apply to you. Each day complete this form to maintain self-support.

Becoming a self-booster:

_____ 1. After I completed my activities during the day, did I notice what I did well while doing them? Did I note what I was proud of, regarding that activity? List three things I did well today that I can take pride in, and review the entire list once per week.
   a.)
   b.)
   c.)

_____ 2. As I was doing different activities, did I complement and praise myself?

_____ 3. Did I take time to savor my accomplishments and feel good about myself?

_____ 4. If I did something not up to my standards or other people's standards, did I give a reason for it, so there is a justification for lower job performance?

_____ 5. Did I avoid evaluating my job performance and criticizing myself? If I did make mistakes doing an activity, did I use descriptive judgments instead to describe how I acted doing a task to learn how to improve performance in the future?

_____ 6. If I determined that a job was not done well, did I give minimum attention to that fact once it was over? Did I avoid getting stuck on negative job performance?

Becoming self-compassionate:

_____ 1. Was I having problems today meeting an expectation of:
   a. an employer _____
   b. my coworkers _____
   c. my spouse or significant other _____
   d. my friends _____
   e. my children _____

_____ 2. Did I excuse myself from meeting that expectation or standard when I could not meet it due to my illness? Did I give myself permission not to do something I could not do?

_____ 3. Did I modify the expectation for myself, by taking into consideration what I cannot do because of my illness?

_____ 4. Did I turn aside guilt for not meeting an expectation?

_____ 5. How much guilt did I feel today about not meeting expectations, from 0 to 100? _____

_____ 6. Did I show myself caring when I could not meet expectations or standards? Did I appear understanding and compassionate to myself when I could not be the way I would like to be?

_____ 7. What acts of self-compassion did I perform today?

Becoming a self-advocate:

_____ 1. Was there a need today to present my side of things or reasons for why I could not or would not perform an action because of my illness? Did I do that?

_____ 2. Did I defend myself when I or other's criticized me for why I did not do something successfully today, because of my illness?

_____ 3. Did I educate others about why I cannot do something, or about how my disease limits what I can do?

_____ 4. Did I set limits on other's behavior toward me if their actions affect me negatively?

_____ 5. Did I set limits in an assertive but not an aggressive way?

_____ 6. Did I feel entitled to speak up or did I feel guilty for doing so?

_____ 7. Did I only hold myself accountable for what I can do within my own area of influence? Did I only focus on what I can do personally?

_____ 8. Did I avoid holding myself responsible for influencing what is outside of my area of influence (what I cannot change personally)?

Self-Esteem Rating: _____

What was my degree of self-esteem today, using the following measure: _____

1 = thought of myself very badly today. Self-esteem very low today.
2 = thought of myself as mildly worthwhile today.
3 = thought of myself as moderately worthwhile today.
4 = thought of myself as very worthwhile today.
5 = thought of myself as most worthwhile. Self-esteem very high today.

TREATMENT OF GUILT

The last three skills focus on how to build positive feelings in the patient. This section covers how to build self-support by removing guilt. As symptoms emerge and limit or preclude role functioning, guilt about disappointing and inconveniencing others is often felt.

Coping with guilt is a major issue in the crisis and post-crisis phases. If guilt is not resolved, it lengthens and intensifies the crises phase. Oppositely, the ability to avoid or expunge guilt about limitations allows patients to move into the synthesis phase.

Cognitive restructuring would focus on absolutistic, unreasonable thinking regarding performance of duties, and would cite it as a primary reason for guilt (Ellis & Abrams, 1994). Imperative thinking would maintain that non-fulfillment of role duties is never permitted, and that those who violate standards for performance are awful. Logical analysis is conducted to counter imperative thinking. It reveals that there are situations where people can be exempted from role responsibilities. To substitute for unreasonable thinking, **relativistic thinking** is stressed. It maintains that role performance and role responsibilities need to be *relative* to the situation. **Anti-imperative thinking** is promoted, such as, "Performing my role duties is preferable but it is not a must."

Patients may also feel guilty because of severe, extreme evaluations of themselves, such as "I am awful or terrible if I disappoint others or cannot satisfy role requirements." Again, relativistic thinking is prescribed along with anti-awfulizing disputation: "Non-performance does cause some problems and is a bad thing, but other factors in life can cause much worse problems. Non-performance is not awful; it is just not desirable. It needs to be seen *relative* to other problems or difficulties." A semantic intervention is then used to show the patient that by using more moderate evaluative words, such as "dislike," a less negative emotion is felt ("I dislike not satisfying role duties but it is not awful if I don't").

If patients reject rational thinking, cognitive restructuring would deal with that by engaging in more disputation. The intent is to gradually chip away at the stubborn allegiance to incorrect thinking. The premise is that deeply ingrained feelings need continued countering of beliefs and in time that will result in emotional change.

CCT uses a method to treat guilt called **exoneration training** that relies on self-questioning. It features a form of cognitive restructuring practiced on the self in an adjudication-type proceeding, along with a paradoxical tactic. The disc contains a worksheet for patients (handout 19) that guides them through the steps in performing this skill.

OTHER SKILLS TO AVOID GUILT AND SELF-BLAME

Another reason for guilt and self-blame is excessive responsibility. Many times people believe that they are legitimately able to be or do something when they are not able to be that way. They need an ability to assess what they are and are not responsible for. This is the skill of **area thinking**.

For example, Julianne has myasthenia gravis. She is upset with how her body looks and feels guilty for not being able to accomplish all of her old responsibilities. Using area thinking, she is able to correct her negative view of self. She wants to look better. She first sets tasks for herself that she can appropriately perform and is able to accomplish. She engages in self-grooming and applying cosmetics at the start of the day to look her best. Second, she determines what is outside of her area of influence and what she cannot accomplish. For instance, she cannot change her expressionless appearance, droopy eyelids, and gaping mouth; they are out of her area of influence. They are symptoms of her disease that she cannot alter. Area thinking sets what she is responsible for regarding role duties. At the start of the day she can perform some actions when she has had a chance to rest her muscles. Area thinking also sets when she is not responsible—at the end of the day when her muscles are weak. Thinking this way she decreases self-blame and guilt.

A second skill to avoid guilt is **entitlement thinking**. Many patients do not believe that they are entitled to do certain actions and thinking that way they feel guilty. They need to reassure themselves about what they are entitled to as a medical patient (e.g., being relieved from a duty they cannot perform). Entitlement thinking also facilitates self-appreciation that is needed for self-boosting.

SUMMARY

Identity adulteration, identity alienation, and identity loss are important treatment issues and each can affect self-esteem. Identity is revealed by identity markers, which capture the essence of who the self is. These markers can be worked with in therapy to preserve self-concept. Others and oneself provide feedback about the patient and that feedback creates images that need to be scrutinized daily. Identity coalescing works to maintain the old identity if it was positive, and integrate it with the new images of self. Self-support skills include self-boosting (focusing on what is done well and minimizing what is not done well), self-compassion (which includes permission giving, mercy, and soft-heartedness), and self-advocacy (which includes educating others, protecting oneself against other's complaints, and justifying one's behavior to others when necessary). To deal with guilt, cognitive restructuring or exoneration training can be utilized.

Chapter 8

Tolerance Skills

It makes sense that medical patients are reluctant to accept their disease. Their body is deviating from the norm for how bodies are supposed to be. Yet, the situation must be tolerated. Many diseases mark patients as different from others and they may even feel disfigured. That too must be tolerated. Because of disease, patients are not able to meet their own or others' standards, but that has to be permitted. In a certain way of thinking, a disease will have its own way with people; it will take control and set the agenda for the day. However, medical patients have to have a capacity and practice that allows for that, taking into consideration the nature of their disease. In summary, chronic and terminal illness patients are forced to withstand many undesirable circumstances and must do so in order to have a satisfactory life.

To be able to do so, they must possess a set of skills that develop the capacity to tolerate such problems as discomfort, frustration, anxiety, rejection, deprivation, and limitation. This chapter focuses on the components of tolerance-based skills. A tolerance skill is part philosophy and part technology.

PHILOSOPHY OF TOLERANCE

Patients can have mental reservations about a disease, but if they have tolerance then they *reluctantly accept* its presence. Acceptance is a coming to terms with the reality that the situation is inescapable. With that in mind, the situation is received into one's life, as part of the usual and customary. This acceptance must occur on an intellectual level, where patients admit what is reality, and on an emotional level, *carry on through the anguish.* Negative feelings are quieted despite hardship as the individual suffers patiently. To do this willingness must be present to co-exist with an unwanted aspect of life. That willingness extends to developing a relationship with the disease, where the patient shows civil and polite behavior toward it. While people obviously do not want to be sick there is resignation that being that way cannot be avoided, which facilitates patience with one's symptoms.

To do this, a decision must be made on a subconscious or conscious level, to withstand and endure. Because the emotional predilection is to damn, hate, and regret illness, to counter that tendency a deliberate determination has to be exerted to practice the mechanics of tolerance (covered in the next section).

Patients may not want to embrace this philosophy, but if they do not they will pay a price for their reluctance, and providers need to educate patients about what is the price. They will end up at war with their pathogen, their disability, their body. They will not find peace-of-mind nor feel at rest with what they are becoming. Without tolerance, the specter of bitterness will continue to hang over them. Hence, for purely practical reasons tolerance with the disease is necessary. Providers need to discuss with patients the utility of tolerance, how it will benefit them. Discuss hatred of disease as an option but also what is lost by being that way. Discuss the benefits of tolerance from a purely selfish standpoint: what the patient will gain by adopting a tolerance perspective.

Before we discuss the specific skills that can facilitate tolerance, there is a need to acquire information about which emotions the patient is having trouble tolerating, what have been troublesome emotions for patients in the past, and what strategies have been used to cope with those emotions. Handout 5 on the disc will identify those feelings.

THE MECHANICS OF TOLERANCE

The following information explains the "how tos" for developing tolerance. By practicing the skills below, medical patients will develop a capacity and procedure for enduring and withstanding disagreeable, distressing situations and emotions.

SELF-MONITORING

Everyone needs to know how much a particular activating event is affecting them. A particular awareness ability is needed, **self-monitoring**. This is an ability to recognize that something is happening and at what level it is occurring. A qualitative measure is too inexact. Self-monitoring is part of self-management therapy (Kanfer, 1970; Rehm & Rokke, 1988; Rokke & Rehm, 2001).

Self-monitoring needs to occur on an on-going basis, whereby people routinely check-in with themselves throughout the day and night to recognize and evaluate their current level of emotion. An example of a time-interval self-monitoring form is provided on the disc (handout 20). It will yield information about the degree of negative emotion during a given time period. The correlation between an emotion and a physical state (e.g., pain, fatigue) can also be tracked. For example, the ratio 4/5 can mean severe level of anger (4) experienced that time period and physical pain (5) during that same time.

Self-monitoring also requires the development of a *shuttling ability,* where patients move back and forth between the activating event and the response to it. This is an awareness capacity to focus on the presenting problem without becoming immersed in it, while at the same time shifting back to attend to the internal response to the problem.

RELAXATION TRAINING

Once there is knowledge of the degree of a negative emotion, the next step is easing the distress and tension contained in the emotion. This involves the ability of *arousal management.* Arousal accompanies such feelings as anxiety, anger, or frustration. It is part of situations where there is rejection or disapproval. Lowering the level of arousal makes it easier to tolerate any of those negative emotions. To do so, providers will teach patients how to slow the rate of breathing and decrease blood pressure, heart rate, and adrenaline. This will involve de-escalating sympathetic functioning or escalating parasympathetic functioning.

Relaxation training facilitates this task (Pelletier, 1977; Poppen, 1988). There are several types of relaxation exercises: deep breathing, progressive muscle relaxation (Jacobson, 1938, 1972), autogenic training (Schultz & Luthe, 1969), guided imagery (Sheikh, 1983), where parts of a scene are seen, heard, and felt (Lang, 1977), and meditation (Benson, 1975; Benson, Beary, & Carol, 1974). While the latter uses a made-up mantra, scheduled, quiet resting may produce similar results (Holmes, 1984). In each exercise, motoric and visceral activities are modified through self-instruction over an extended time period.

The disc contains a handout (number 21) describing these relaxation exercises. They require several minutes of time (10–15 minutes) and should become a regular part of the medical patient's day. Set-up a self-evaluation form to assess if relaxation is being done.

There are many situations, though, where medical patients do not have time to leave the troublesome situation and go off to relax for an extended time period. They only have seconds available to de-escalate arousal while still participating in the situation. In that case, quick relaxation techniques are necessary. Examples of several of them are provided on handout 22 on the disc. These techniques combine elements of traditional relaxation techniques. Providers will need to work with patients to de-focus off of the upsetting foreground image and make a neutral or positive image foreground in its place. This is part of Gestalt management discussed below.

After patients have had time to acquire the habit of self-monitoring and have learned basic relaxation ability, use cognitive rehearsal training to further develop those skills. They would imagine being in a difficult situation, monitoring how upset the fantasy makes them feel, and then use relaxation to become calm, as Wolpe (1958) recommends. Evaluate the level of arousal after completing each relaxation exercise. This should be practiced several times a day.

To increase facility in becoming relaxed in difficult, physically arousing situations, *systematic desensitization* can be employed (Wolpe, 1973). This is a covert conditioning procedure where patients categorize events and actions that cause autonomic arousal in increasing order of difficulty. Each activity is imagined and a relaxation technique is used when arousal occurs.

GESTALT MANAGEMENT

Gestalt therapy makes the point that one's focus of attention sharply influences what is felt. Perceiving negative matters will cause negative emotions. Once something becomes foreground that will naturally increase energy and motivation to change the situation (Perls, Hefferline, & Goodman, 1951; Polster & Polster, 1973). By focusing on negative matters there will be less hope and more pessimism about changing the situation (Snyder, Cheavens, & Micheal, 1999). Hence, one way to tolerate a difficult situation is by managing what is foreground and what will be the composition of the background.

This is termed **Gestalt management**, which is the process of deliberately selecting foreground images against a background and together they comprise a Gestalt. There are various techniques in positioning a desirable foreground image. The disc contains a handout on two of them: sensory diversion training (handout 23) and psychological distancing (handout 23). The Coping Skills Book details three other techniques: no-mind-no thing, proximal thinking, and thought stopping.

MIND-SET FOR TOLERANCE

The above techniques will help but they will not work nearly as well unless there is a change in thinking about how to relate to the disease and the treatment for it. Three mind-sets will become crucial: a) self-assurance that tolerance is possible, b) acceptance of challenge to tolerate, and c) acceptance of the problem. Each becomes part of a person's self-talk. Each need to become part of the executive beliefs for developing a tolerance skill.

Developing Self-Assurance

If patients consider their disease to be intolerable then they believe that there is no way they can live with their condition. If they believe that they lack internal support—coping ability—to bear their situation, then they will assume that their disease exceeds reasonable limits of endurance. In that case, they will maintain that they will not be able to co-exist with their physical condition. The only way out is removal of what cannot be removed. This places patients in an untenable situation.

But so much of tolerance has to do with one's view of self. People can tolerate a highly difficult situation if they believe that they are capable of enduring. That is a precondition to willingness to take on the challenge of enduring. People will put their mind on coping if they believe that they are capable of doing so. This has to do with the issue of self-assurance: to know that you have what it takes to succeed.

How can a therapist convince a patient of this? In part this can be accomplished by a solution-oriented approach (de Shazer, 1985, 1988, 1991; O'Hanlon & Weiner-Davis, 1989). There are times when people do tolerate their troublesome situation better than other times. They may assume tolerance is impossible, that their physical condition or the problems it causes (e.g., excessive frustration) are "too much." But in most cases incapacity is not steady. There are times when there are exceptions to incapacity; there is not always the same level of non-success. When there is greater tolerance that constitutes an "exception moment." It refutes the patient's unrealistic hypothesis that tolerance is impossible. Therefore, providers can:

1). Have patients focus on exception moments, and what they did to contribute to a positive outcome. This is important when exception moments are occurring but patients are not sure how it happened. Inquire, "How did you manage to take this important step to cope with _____?, or "What were you telling yourself to get ready to cope with _____?" This helps patients realize that they were unconsciously working to tolerate problems. It reinforces that the individual is capable of bearing difficulty (White & Epston, 1988). Ask the patient why things are not worse if they presume that they cannot cope ("What are you doing to keep yourself from feeling even more overwhelmed by _____ (e.g., all of your anxieties about your future)?" This reassures patients that they actually have coping capacity without conscious awareness of its existence (Berg & Gallagher, 1991).

2) Ask a percentage question (de Shazer, 1985, 1991; Selekman, 1999): "What percentage of the time do you have more success managing _____ (e.g., your daily deprivations?"). This increases awareness of exception moments.

3) After finding out how much of the time there is a lack of tolerance of difficult situations, inquire what the patient will have to do to raise tolerance 10%, and then 20%, and so on. This is referred to as a scaling question (de Shazer, 1985, 1991). It creates the idea of change in small steps.

4). Have the patient predict—before beginning his or her day—if that day will be a coping or non-coping day and then observe if the prediction turns out to be true (Berg & Miller, 1992; Miller & Berg, 1995).

5) Have the patient flip a coin if the next day will be a miracle day, when the difficult situation is not a problem (e.g., uncertainty is not causing the person a problem). Then have the patient follow the predetermined course the coin told him/her to take (Miller & Berg, 1995).

A second way to treat faith in one's incapacity to tolerate is by dealing with that way of thinking as non-utilitarian thinking. Believing the self lacks capacity to tolerate decreases motivation to practice tolerance skills. Without practice there is a lack of evidence that the self is capable of enduring negative emotions. This results in a lack of self-assurance, which subsequently causes an increase in anxiety about having a medical problem. Hence, believing in an inability to tolerate leads to greater distress. Use cognitive restructuring to challenge this idea.

Patients need to understand that tolerance is not an all-or-nothing matter. Some patients think dichotomously: "I've got this ability or I don't have it." Instead, reassure patients that tolerance is acquired incrementally. Have the patient estimate each day *how much* she can possibly raise her tolerance limits, from 0 to 100, with 100 being total success at coping with an unwanted condition (e.g., disapproval and rejection from others). Then, the next day, raise tolerance a little bit more, and so on.

Accepting Challenge to Tolerate

Often, people confuse the challenge to tolerate with the ability to tolerate. The latter actually involves identity—if someone believes that he or she has or does not have tolerance potential. The former refers to the activity of activating skills for management. It also refers to the degree of difficulty that exists in the quest to succeed at tolerance. With more challenge there will be varying degrees of success at tolerance but that is different from not possessing the ability at all.

The treatment task is getting patients to assume the challenge of tolerating and having faith and confidence that it can be achieved. An attitude needs to be developed—through self-dialogue—to motivate patients to enter the contest to achieve some degree of tolerance capacity.

Self-instruction training can develop this ability. Below is a boilerplate self-dialogue (handout 25 on disc) that can be used to buoy willingness to take on the challenge of tolerance. Simply substitute the situation the patient faces (e.g., rejection, on-going personal limitations, frequent disappointments) for the letter X.

HANDOUT 8.1: Self-talk to Develop Tolerance***

Preparing for a challenge:
I have to face X and that will test my ability to cope.

It is a challenge but I have faced this challenge before and have succeeded.

Do not be intimidated by the challenge to tolerate this situation.

I do not have to be 100% successful. I just have to make the situation bearable to a greater degree.

I can tolerate X if I put my mind to it. Believe in myself.

I feel overwhelmed by X at this moment. I do not think I can tolerate it right now.

Only reduce X by 20% right now. Set a realistic goal for what I can tolerate.

Do not be a black-and-white thinker. Do not think in terms of total tolerance or total incapacity.

Take on the challenge to manage. Do not back-off. I can accomplish what is reasonable.

Work at coping. Build up to adjusting. It will not happen immediately. Take small steps.

Do not set a goal of total eradication of X. It won't happen. Do not disappoint myself by thinking unrealistically.

Do a relaxation exercise. De-focus from what's stressful.

For other examples of self-dialogues, the disc contains handouts for patients to develop their ability to tolerate helplessness (handout 26), frustration (handout 27), disfigurement (handout 28), disappointment (handout 29), and uncertainty (handout 30). In addition, there are worksheets to train patients in how to relate to risk (handout 31) and how to perform problem-solving (handout 32), so uncertainty can be tolerated easier.

ACCEPTANCE OF PROBLEM

A primary reason patients dislike the problem that they face is because of absolutistic thinking such as, "My life should not include X (e.g., unpredictable and uncertain situations) or not have so much of Y (e.g., pain, helplessness)." Absolutistic thinking indicates unwillingness to accept the problem situation. Instead, thinking needs to be reformulated *to allow for the problem situation and to accept it* because it cannot be avoided. Self-instruction training is helpful for that purpose. The self-dialogue instructs patients in how to respond to gain acceptance.

HANDOUT 8.2: *Self-talk for Problem Situations*

I cannot have control in this situation.

It's unpleasant having X but I can bear it if I work on it to some degree.

Accept the fact that my life will contain X.

Don't hate that fact.

I don't know when X will not be part of my life. I'd like to know but I don't have to know in order to be content.

In the meantime, while X is present in my life, I need to work on tolerating it.

It would be nice to know how my life will be in the future but I don't have that information. Accept that.

I can still have control, though, by practicing tolerance skills. Control what I can control, especially my own responses to X.

I can make alternative plans and be happy if I know how to tolerate this unpleasant situation. Tolerance gives me freedom.

Stay in the here-and-now. Deal with the problem facing me right now and learn how to bear it. That I can control.

I would like to be without X but I can work to overcome it behaviorally.

In the meantime deal with what I am facing this moment. I have to tolerate its presence. It would be nice not to have X but that is not my situation.

Living a life with X is not desirable but it is not awful either. I make things awful when I hate having X in my life.

The self-dialogue has several missions.

1) Gain acceptance of the present problem. That is an internal matter.
2) At the same time the dialogue frees patients to behaviorally change the situation.
3) Gain acceptance of uncertainty about how long that problem will be a factor in people's lives. Develop an appropriate attitude about uncertainty, that it is not the worst thing facing a person.
4) Build tolerance to facilitate capacity to suffer. Once achieved, the problem no longer controls the patient. Tolerance frees the patient from the problem. It may still exist but its impact is diminished. This automatically changes the evaluation of the problem, so it is not conceptualized as awful any longer.

ROLE MODEL ENACTMENT

Another way to increase tolerance is by becoming someone else who is capable of being tolerant. This is termed *role model enactment* (Sharoff, 2004). Inquire if patients know anyone who can cope with the problem that they face (e.g., extensive uncertainty in their life). That person can then become the patient's role model in this one regard. After identifying the role model, inquire how that person is able to cope with his or her problem. The intention is to increase curiosity about how the role model functions, and then copy that approach.

An alternative idea is to make a group of people a role model. Inquire about groups of people who regularly face a problem in their life. The problem may be due to where they live or a historical circumstance. For instance, if the problem is increasing uncertainty, there were times when people faced uncertainty due to economic problems such as in the Great Depression or during international struggles. In each case those people had to learn tactics to live with unpredictability. Again, the focus shifts to how they psychologically survived in such circumstances. If the problem is rejection by others, inquire how groups of people who have been rejected (e.g., Jews, African-Americans) coped with that problem.

REFRAMING

Another way to treat the existence of a problem is by seeing it from a different perspective. Instead of viewing it as all bad it can be redefined as beneficial in some way. This switch in viewpoint makes it easier to tolerate any problem. This is facilitated by the tactic of *reframing*. In this technique, patients are asked to list the pros and cons, the problems and benefits to having that troublesome event or feeling in their life. For instance, if people face routine deprivation due to their disease, can that benefit them at some point in their life, such as when they have to move into retirement and have to live without as much money as when they were working.

SUMMARY

Tolerance is an ability to withstand a negative situation or negative emotion. A philosophy is in part necessary to gain acceptance of tolerance as a strategy. The philosophy maintains that an unpleasant stimulus can be accepted if it cannot be eradicated, and that there must be a willingness to co-exist with it. What is unpleasant will create distress, so there must be awareness of how much distress is present. This requires the ability of self-monitoring. Next, the negative stimulus creates arousal, so relaxation is necessary to lower arousal. An effort must be made to focus on other matters to reduce the impact of the negative stimulus. A mindset is most important for tolerance. It includes developing self-assurance that the negative stimulus can be endured, and acceptance of the challenge to tolerate. Self-instruction will guide the development of tolerance ability. Other methods to build tolerance include role model enactment, outcome enactment, and reframing.

Chapter 9

Accommodation Skills

The last chapter dealt with how to withstand a negative situation. This chapter deals with ***how to withstand a recurring negative situation***, such as frequent disappointment, unavoidable deprivation and frustration, anxiety that will not go away, or repeated rejection. When there is a recurring negative emotion, quite often a counter reaction occurs. There is frustration about being frustrated too much of the time, rejection of routine disapproval, anxiety about having another anxiety attack, or disappointment about suffering through another round of disappointments. In such an environment enthusiasm to tolerate problems wanes and a demand is made for an end to such a circumstance. But when that demand cannot be met that only adds to the feeling of impotency. This contributes to two derivative consequences: brooding and mental castigation of forces that seem to maintain the situation, such as the disease itself, God, life, or medical personnel.

The problem of recurring negative events is a basic and common dilemma facing medical patients. They have to choose how to respond to it. One option is engaging in absolutistic thinking and commanding life to be different. This means the patient is internally at war with his or her health care problem or whomever is causing the negative feeling to continue. But that battle will prove futile and cause more problems in the long-term, because the problem will remain in effect. The patient is battling something that cannot be eradicated—their disease and its consequences. Another option is ***accommodation to the unwanted condition***. That response will yield numerous benefits, such as peace-of-mind and better adjustment to disease and treatment. This chapter focuses on the accommodation response and how to develop it in medical patients.

THE ACCOMMODATION RESPONSE

CCT defines accommodation as an internal activity and not a behavior. It is what people do inside themselves when they face a situation that is not liked or wanted. What are the components of accommodation?

1) Recognition of reality: to know intellectually and emotionally what has to be faced because that is the present prevailing truth.
2) Allowance of reality, whatever it may be: to let something happen or permit it. While disease will happen whether the individual allows it or not, he does have a choice in how he responds to it. He can protest, disallow and reject reality or concede that it will occur and permit its presence. By doing so, the individual does not lose his position and can still dislike and disapprove of his situation, but he is not engaged in active protest.
3) Integrate the disease into his life: This makes the medical patient a whole human being again and no longer someone alienated from a dominant part of himself—his diseased body. "I have two arms, two legs, two eyes, and X (e.g., chronic pain, fatigue, weakness, etc.). The disease then becomes one part, albeit a major part, of who the self is.
4) Co-exist with the disease: Room is made for the disease—within oneself—for the unpleasant, discomforting physical sensations, adverse consequences, and limitations. Essentially, *accommodation is the act of containment.* Containment in this context does not mean to suppress or "keep a lid on" feelings, but to make room for something within. When practiced adeptly, accommodation allows patients to hold the many negative changes in their life comfortably within themselves.

Let us compare the accommodation response to non-accommodation. The latter is detected by such statements as, "I've had it. I don't want this anymore. I want this out of my life." There is unwillingness to let anymore of that negative emotion exist within oneself, and **refusal to integrate the consequences of disease** (e.g., further disappointments or rejection). No room is being made for an unwanted entity (e.g., death, disability, medical incompetence, or medical incapacity) to exist within one's life, psyche, or body. Basically, non-accommodation means a declaration of war against the present reality.

Oppositely, accommodation stops viewing disease and its consequences as the enemy and instead views it as an unwanted facet or feature of self. Accommodation overcomes the urge to disallow disease. It is not an act of conceding to a greater power but an act of making peace with that power. By being willing to co-exist with one's physical condition, brooding and castigation of the disease and whoever supposedly caused the disease (e.g., oneself, employer, God, poor medical care) ceases. Hence, accommodation allows the patient to transcend his situation.

For instance, when disappointments commonly occur, accommodation will make room for them. Likewise, when deprivation cannot be avoided and is mandated by one's situation, accommodation is practiced to ease frustration about that. If rejection continues to occur, accommodation helps by forging realization that is part of one's lot in life. If a patient constantly feels helpless, accommodation helps him grow used to a lack of control.

Discuss with patients what they have to gain by pursuing accommodation. First, it facilitates Gestalt management. When patients lack accommodation they continuously think about their troubles, their disease, and all the problems it has brought. This causes negative matters to remain foreground and pushes good tidings in life and potential positive developments into the background. Oppositely, accommodation integrates the disease and its consequences into the person's life. They become part of the background, one of the many aspects of the self, which allows positive matters to become foreground and appreciated all the more. When the focus is no longer on responding to troubles, energy can then be shifted to finding new sources of meaning. That builds thankfulness for what the patient has instead of focusing on what has been lost. The penalties from having disease are not abhorred nearly as much because the patient makes peace with them and allows them to exist within. This all creates a measure of good will, the feeling of grace. From a general health standpoint, accommodation aids the physical war on disease because it eases distress that depletes the immune system (Selye, 1976). It eases neuromuscular activity, which will ease physical pain. Accommodation will cause patients to decrease utilization of the health care system. They will live with problems instead of trying to eradicate them via further testing and doctor visits.

DEVELOPING THE MIND-SET OF ACCOMMODATION

Let us now examine the role of cognition in developing accommodation. While problems differ there are common executive beliefs and self-instructions necessary for building an accommodation response. The disc contains a model self-dialogue to develop accommodation ability (handout 33). The disc also contains self-dialogues on accommodating to deprivation (handout 35), bodily changes (handout 36), and rejection (handout 37). To further explicate how to build the thought structure underpinning accommodation, a self-dialogue is presented below on the subject of unavoidable helplessness (see handout 9.1 below). Notice the following main ideas in the self-dialogue: (a) Integrate the unwanted reality that a negative emotion will persist or recur; (b) Reaffirm capacity to cope with that reality; (c) Surrender the protest against reality because it will do no good; (d) Realize that negative feelings do not have to feel awful once they are accepted as part of one's lot in life; (e) Focus on what can be controlled, what is within one's area of influence.

HAND-OUT 9.1: Helplessness Allowance Training***

Preparing for being unable to control how the body acts or feels:

I cannot control how my body is doing. This is the way it is right now. Accept that. Live with it.

Give up my anger about not being able to make my body feel the way I want it to.

Be ready to feel helpless when my body does not respond as I want it to.

I cannot control how my body will be, feel, and act, except by complying with the medical regimen. What I can control I will work on.

When my body does not perform as I want I will accept that fact.

My disease has made many changes in my life and I am helpless to change those changes. Accommodate to that fact. Allow helplessness in when it cannot be avoided.

Don't get into thinking that it is a must that my body perform as I want.

Must" means of the utmost importance and controlling my body is not of the utmost importance—it is only preferable that I control my body.

I can still find happiness even if I cannot control my body.

Managing my resentment when I am helpless:

I am falling into anger with my helplessness.

How much anger do I feel right now from 0 to 5, with 5 being enraged?

Relax. Breathe deeply. Being tense does not help.

I am demanding that I not be helpless when that is not possible. I am fighting against accepting reality. Let reality into my life.

I am refusing to accept my body as it is. I have decided not to contain my disappointment in what I have become.

That will only make me feel worse. Do I want to feel worse?

Let the helplessness into my life. I can live with it, even though I don't like being that way. I can make it part of me, if I choose.

I will accommodate to the loss of the ability to control my body.

I will accommodate to the changes brought by my disease. I am helpless to prevent those changes. That I must accept.

TREATING RESISTANCE

Providers will often encounter resistance to the idea of accommodation because it goes against the basic need for enhancement and reward: people naturally want the best situation for themselves. There are several causes for resistance. The coping skills approach for treating resistance to accommodation is discussed.

BELIEFS CAUSING RESISTANCE

A. *Unrealistic Thinking*

Patients resist accommodation to the disease when they maintain that their life should not have that particular problem (e.g. frequent disappointment). Behind this belief is demandingness or insistence that things be different. CCT deals with the protest against reality as a coping response and then examines the viability of that response ("Will protest make you feel better?"). **Constructive mourning** (Sharoff, 2002, 2004) is suggested to address underlying sadness about that undesirable situation. **Area thinking** is tried to refocus the patient on what he or she can change. **Tolerance** techniques are suggested to ease discomfort from the negative situation. Then, the accommodation response is promoted and worked on using several different methods, such as self-instruction training, imagery, symbolic gesturing, or other measures (see Coping Skills Book for details). The CR approach would convert the imperative belief into a hypothesis and collect evidence to show that the undesirable situation cannot be avoided. The tendency for demandingness is countered. Adaptive thinking is then emphasized for coping purposes ("I would like things to be different but they are not that way.").

B. Extreme, Unrealistic Evaluations

Patients resist accommodation because it is viewed as terrible or awful. CCT would go along with the patient's viewpoint if he rigorously adheres to this perspective. The emphasis would shift to coping with an awful situation. Effort would be on building self-assurance that an awful situation can be managed, using such measures as **self-support training**, building an identity of a coping person (e.g., through identity markers), and **discomfort tolerance training** (Sharoff, 2004). This compares to the CR approach that would inculcate relativistic thinking: "You have a bad situation but compare it to others." While this puts the patient's situation into perspective and creates greater objectivity, it does not train coping responses.

C. Demandingness

Patients resist accommodation because they choose to order an undesirable situation out of their life. They pursue a mission to eradicate the problem and not adjust to it. CCT believes this belief is perpetuated by an agonistic tendency, a tendency to battle against something until it is changed. The treatment for this is discussed in chapter 10.

LETTING GO

Another basic reason patients resist accommodation is because they do not want to accept the loss of what could have been—their dreams, goals, and hopes of a different and better life. In essence, they do not want to let go of who they were, where they were heading, and what they could have had if their disease did not enter their life. Even though the facts may show that they cannot return to who they were they still fight that determination.

This is due to an agonistic tendency to battle to salvage a former self, lifestyle, and future. That struggle does not have to be problematic *if* there is hope of reclaiming the lost self. In that case patients should be told to do behaviorally what is necessary to heal themselves. While they are doing so they only have to practice tolerance of a present situation that in time will be corrected.

The issue of not letting go is more complicated when patients have little hope of a cure, that the condition will be lasting or deadly. In that case providers can discuss the pros and cons of maintaining a strategy that fights against adjustment. Second, providers can still recommend doing what can be done behaviorally to change the situation, as long as the patient internally accepts the prevailing reality that at that point in time accommodation is necessary.

If the medical situation cannot be corrected, though, providers will need to promote acceptance of reality. That often leads to a grief reaction about losing the former self or lifestyle due to disease. CCT would then encourage the use of **constructive mourning** as a bereavement tool (Sharoff, 2002, 2004) for that purpose.

Two other factors will need to be addressed to encourage letting go. One, providers will need to show patients that they can achieve some measure of a satisfying life, even with their disease. This leads to the task of **meaning-making** (see Coping Skills Book for discussion of this activity). A second issue is the need for **limitation accommodation** (see Sharoff, 2004, for fuller discussion). For instance, there may be limits on mobility, how much approval can be achieved from others, or limits on pursuing premorbid activities. Treatment will involve the need for **body accommodation** and **disfigurement neutralization** (see Coping Skills Book). Providers will need to build a mindset that accepts limits imposed by the disease and treatment. Entailed in this is recognition of what cannot be changed and achieved, which involves the need for area thinking.

SELF-PITY RESCUE

Some patients resist accommodation because it goes against their basic way of comforting themselves when they are penalized or feel at a loss. That basic way involves the use of self-pity. Self-pity is compassion given to oneself but it takes the form of feeling sorry for oneself. It is a descent into "woe is me" thinking, by characterizing oneself as a victim or poor soul. Thinking this way portrays the disease or whoever contributes to problems as bad and harmful. In a roundabout way, self-pity is a poor form of grieving about having to endure an unwanted situation. Behind self-pity is absolutistic thinking, which rules that life be different than how it presently is. Also behind self-pity is a subtle demand for another outcome (e.g., no more deprivation, less disappointment). The problem with self-pity is that it actually stimulates more resentment and bitterness and leads to depression, because it conceptualizes the person's life pejoratively.

To treat this problem, providers need to raise patients' awareness that they engage in this pastime. Next, self-pity is categorized as a coping strategy. The pros and cons of this strategy are then discussed, so patients understand what they gain and lose by using it. At the same time the positive aspects of self-pity need to be preserved, such as self-concern and self-compassion. However, the form of self-compassion in self-pity needs to be modified, because it overemphasizes misfortune, bad luck, and disfavor by super-powerful forces like fate, contagion, God, or HMOs. It characterizes patients as weak by seeing them as victims.

In opposition to that patients need to be taught a healthy form of self-compassion, which extends aid and support without feeling sorry for oneself. Patients are taught to acknowledge their feelings (e.g., "It hurts me not being able to do what I enjoy") without resorting to regressive, child-like ways of expressing grief (e.g., withdrawal, whining).

Self-instruction training is helpful for avoiding self-pity and pulling oneself out of it when it occurs. The disc contains a self-dialogue (handout 40) that uses relapse-prevention theory. The dialogue prepares patients to cope with difficult situations where they may slip back into a self-pity mode.

RESILIENCY TRAINING

Another reason patients do not embrace accommodation is because they feel overwhelmed. Encountering the effects of disease, they sink into depression or psychological collapse and cannot extricate themselves from it. They feel overpowered by the forces of disease, the exigencies of treatment, and the frustrations of dealing with immense institutions like insurance companies and hospitals. These are patients who lack resilience.

Yet, resilience can be inculcated and developed. Patients need to first set realistic, achievable goals. This is facilitated by *value clarification*, which will detail what is most important to the individual, and *area thinking*, which will detail what can be accomplished by the person himself. *Problem solving* selects what is the best way to accomplish the goal, by using *alternative solution thinking* to identify options. Self-talk needs to buoy spirits and belief in self as capable, which is part of *self-assurance training*. The positive qualities of the patient need to be foreground so there is self-confidence to make attempts to be different, and that is a function of *self-support training*. Finally, self-instructions are used to guide responses to overcome the overwhelmed condition. Below is a self-dialogue*** that summons the above coping skills.

HAND-OUT 9.2: *Self-Talk to Become Resilient*

Preparing for a situation that lowers my spirits:

I have felt down in this situation before. Get ready because it may happen again.
Self-monitor how I feel in the situation so I do not suddenly feel overwhelmed. Do not let it sneak up on me.
Be ready to boost my spirits with reassurance that I can make the situation better. I can make things improve. I can manage.
I do not have to feel overwhelmed and overpowered. I can be tough and in control of my feelings.
Think of times when I managed this same situation in the past. Focus on what I did well in those situations.

Self-talk when feeling overpowered:

Do not get bowled over. That will not do.
Challenge myself to push on. Be a good soldier. March on.
Believe in myself. I can cope with this.
Think of my alternatives in this situation. How can I get the best for myself? Put a plan into effect.
Deal with the problem—do not get overwhelmed by it.
Think of what I need to do next. Take one step at a time.
I feel beaten down now but I do not have to stay that way. What are my strengths? Focus on them.

When implementing the dialogue, markers will need to be declared that reveal the subtle indications of an emerging, overwhelmed feeling. This can be the feeling of being dispirited, slopping shoulders, or sagging chin. On-going self-monitoring will reveal those markers.

Two other approaches are helpful to achieve resilience. Anchoring can be used (King, Novik, & Citrenbaum, 1983), where patients remember times when they rallied and managed under pressure, and those memories are linked to a particular body part. When needing to feel resilient, that body part is touched again to re-fire those potent memory traces. Solution-oriented therapy can also be used (de Shazer, 1985, 1988, 1991). Patients are not always being overwhelmed. There are many times when they cope during the week and need to be aware of that. How they then coped on those occasions becomes the solution for future situations.

SUMMARY

Accommodation seeks a realistic acceptance of what is unwanted but cannot be avoided. It wants patients to integrate what is unwanted into their life and co-exist with it. Self-instruction training helps this effort. People often resist accommodation. Their thinking about it can be restructured when that happens. They may also resist because of a need not to hold on to their dreams for the future, a tendency for self-pity, and an inability to be resilient. Treatment for these issues is presented.

Treatment of Bitterness

This chapter covers one of the most difficult cases for health care providers, the patient embittered about how his life has gone. This group of patients is often not interested in adjustment to their situation, so they resist using what providers have to offer to help them. Instead they seek to undo their situation and make it go away. Moving these patients beyond their anger about how their life has gone or will go is frequently quite difficult.

To a degree, virtually all medical patients show some degree of bitterness. That is because disease takes away what people value. Disease changes lives and forces people to adapt to situations that are not wanted. When enough has been taken, when too many forced changes have been made, the feeling of bitterness arises and hardens.

Bitterness is a mental pain, a state of anguish, torment, and agitation. It includes regret and sorrow mixed with anger, resentment, and indignation about being wronged. Behind those feelings is a belief about unfair treatment that causes the embittered to feel afflicted and aggrieved. In medical patients, there is also disenchantment that beloved ideals for themselves, their life, and their future will not be met (e.g., "I was supposed to retire and golf everyday but now I can hardly get around."). Realizing their ideal existence will not occur, or they will not remain the kind of person that they have always valued, the feeling of bitterness suffuses through their activities. Sharoff (2004) has referred to this as "dream crush," the ending of a cherished idea or fantasy. Before moving on to discuss how to treat bitterness, a questionnaire is provided to measure how much patients feel that way.

---

*Am I Bitter?****

Check off if any of the following apply to you.

_____ 1. It is not right what has happened to me.
_____ 2. Others do not have to go through what I have had to go through.
_____ 3. I often feel like crying or screaming.
_____ 4. I have so much negative feeling pushed down inside of me.
_____ 5. Others have said I am bitter about what has happened to my life.
_____ 6. I often think, "Why me? Why have I been picked out for this grief?"
_____ 7. I think about my misfortunes a lot.
_____ 8. Others seem to get the help they need from others to make them happy but not me.
_____ 9. Often I find myself churning inside.
_____ 10. Life has been a great disappointment to me.
_____ 11. Why can't I get my way like others seem to get their way.
_____ 12. I know what can make me happy but I cannot have it.
_____ 13. Just when I got my hopes built up that things are going to work out for me everything comes crashing down.
_____ 14. I have been let down so many times.
_____ 15. I often feel tense and uptight.
_____ 16. Others have gotten the breaks in life but not me.
_____ 17. I often have thoughts about how things could have gone much better for me.

_____ 18. I see others happy and getting what they want in life and I think, "I should be that way."
_____ 19. Why do others seem to have it all when I have had so much go wrong for me.
_____ 20. Nothing seems to go my way.
_____ 21. When I come down to it, I am just plain mad about how things have gone for me in my life.
_____ 22. I am sick and tired of not being able to do what can make me happy.
_____ 23. Life, God, fate, or luck have not been fair to me.
_____ 24. It is hard keeping my anger from coming out.

Add up the number of checks and if you have more than half checked-off then you may want to consider if you feel bitter about how your life has gone.

In having patients complete the above form, there are five variables that are being measured:

Belief in receiving unfair treatment: 1, 6, 16, 23

Envy: 2, 8, 11, 18, 19

Suppressed anger: 3, 4, 9, 15, 24

Self-pity: 5, 7, 12, 17, 20, 22

Disappointment: 10, 13, 14, 21

Let us now turn our attention to two theories for why there is bitterness. One is based on cognitive restructuring practice theory and the other is from CCT.

COGNITIVE RESTRUCTURING PERSPECTIVE

From the standpoint of REBT, demandingness is a major reason for bitterness (Dryden & Ellis, 1988, 2001; Ellis & Abrams, 1994). When the capacity to tolerate misfortune and crises has been reached, there is a tendency in people to demand no more grief and problems. When the demand is not met the situation is related to as awful, and that belief makes the situation all the harder to tolerate, thus resulting in disenchantment and the sense of being wronged. The imperative thought inflates the _direness_ of the situation in the mind of the individual, causing it to be seen as dreadful, which in turn causes a more intense, negative affect such as bitterness.

REBT counters patient thinking that the situation is awful with the idea that virtually no situation or outcome is truly awful; worse can always be found. Further, no outcome is deemed imperative because virtually no outcome is vital. Vital means crucial—above all else—but situations can always be found that are _more_ crucial (Ellis & Abrams, 1994). In place of imperative thinking, milder evaluations are sought, such as conceptualizing the situation as unfortunate or undesirable, and by doing so milder negative feelings are felt.

(As a practical word of caution, when using CR with medical patients, practitioners may be forced to play with words to encourage patients to surrender their absolutistic thinking. The condition they steadfastly label as awful may have to be relabeled as "highly, highly undesirable" to gain patients' cooperation in changing their thinking. The essential point is still made, though, that the medical patient's situation is bad, but just not as bad as he presumed.)

CCT also agrees that demandingness and awfulizing play a role in the development of bitterness. However, _CCT maintains that the cognitive restructuring position over-simplifies the situation._ CR ignores the role of other variables interacting with absolutistic thinking and awfulizing. It incorrectly presumes that incorrect, irrational thinking accounts for a major amount of the variance in patient behavior and outcome. CCT argues that imperative thinking and awfulizing do not have to lead to a more intense negative affect *if* other variables are not present. In that case the harmful effects from unrealistic, irrational thinking can be greatly minimized.

AN IRRATIONAL, MALADAPTIVE COPING SKILL

What are those other variables mentioned above? What is the coping skills perspective on bitterness? According to CCT, behavior grows out of an interaction of variables that CCT terms an *irrational, maladaptive coping skill*. It is what "*awfulizes*" a situation in the patient's mind (Sharoff, 2002). Let us now examine those variables.

A.   *Tendency for Extreme Evaluative Ratings*

CCT does agree with CR theory that extreme, severe evaluations of a situation (e.g., "losing my health is terrible") are problematic. Evaluating situations in extreme ways does cause people to feel worse when the so-called awful outcome comes to pass. Extreme evaluations do incite, make people reject a situation, and cause unnecessary worry and undue pessimism. It increases the push to disallow the disease.

B.   *Insistence*

Demandingness, or what CCT prefers to call insistence, does lead to inflexibility and difficulty adjusting to unwanted situations. It pushes people to only accept the demanded outcome and no other, so when the prized outcome is not realized there is greater frustration. This way of thinking transcends the limited capacity of people in an effort to seize control when that is not possible.

CCT concedes that awfulizing and absolutistic thinking certainly lead to difficulties, but asserts that their impact can be short-lived and limited in duration, providing the other variables discussed below are not present. If the variables below are present, then they will escalate and inflame negative emotion and cause awfulizing and insistent thinking to be far more virulent.

Severe, negative evaluations and imperative thinking are both beliefs. The variables may arise from how people think but they also can be due to other factors as well, such as trauma, personality structure, genetic predisposition, early life conditioning, and conscious, determined choice.

C.   *Agonistic Tendency*

This is a tendency to strive to overcome obstacles, brush aside handicaps, resist others, pursue unwanted actions, and combat forces perceived as hostile to one's interests. The agonistic nature strains to achieve a desired outcome. It is a willingness to contest, not to take "no" for an answer. It stirs motivation. It summons arguments and reasons for why something should and must occur (or not occur). It channels energy into a struggle to gain what is wanted and avoid the unwanted. It will use absolutistic thinking to provide the content for its position, but it does not have to arise from thinking.

The agonistic nature can function as either an adaptive or a maladaptive coping response. It can be beneficial or harmful depending on the context in which it is used and how it is used. For instance, it is adaptive in terminal illness when it pushes patients to live on when their body is failing. In chronic illness patients, it is the force that turns them into "good soldiers" who march on when their body aches or cannot easily move. On the other hand, it can cause patients to persevere in ideation that resists reality. If genetically caused, the agonistic tendency appears early in a child's life as perseverance, oppositional-defiant behavior, perfectionism, or overly persistent and conscientious traits. It is what makes some children exacting and copious hard workers who strive to achieve in academics or sports. If caused by trauma, it can produce anxious, stubborn unwillingness to alter a feared course.

Both absolutistic thinking and awfulizing interact with the agonistic tendency, where each influences the other. Irrational, unrealistic thinking can "hook" an agonistic person to pick up the struggle to battle on to gain one's position or a cherished outcome. Oppositely, the driven nature to combat can make a person think in terms of commands and demands. The agonistic tendency provides the energy and continued willfulness to realize the absolutistic thinking. When not getting one's way, the agonistic tendency will view that situation as awful. Oppositely, exaggerating the direness of a situation by viewing it as awful will arouse the agonistic tendency to push to change it.

Without the presence of an agonistic nature, imperative thinking can be put aside or extinguished without an extensive battle. This is why some patients readily change their thinking early in therapy, when presented with a rational counter-argument. Many people have imperative thinking and engage in demandingness and awfulizing, but quickly change with the aid of self-reflection, by discovering contrary facts to their position, or when under pressure from family or friends to think differently. Compare them, though, to agonistic individuals who cling to their ideation in therapy and elsewhere. They withstand pressure from others to think differently, and refute or ignore contrary data not supporting their thinking.

D. Brooding

There are some people who respond to the inability to attain an end-goal with a combination of resentful protest, gloom, sour grapes, sulking, and self-pity. That comprises the brooding response. The brooding tendency can be the result of imperative thinking, but it can also be due to genetic predisposition. Brooding can be a learned response. Parents can condition it when they disallow assertive behavior but reward their children when they act moody and sulk when not getting their way. Brooding can be due to trauma, where a person cannot put aside a searing incident from his or her past.

Absolutistic thinking does not always cause people to brood. There are some absolutistic thinkers who do not engage in brooding, so when they insist on something happening and it does not occur they can move on without slipping into a dark, dismal mood. Likewise, there are agonistic individuals who are not prone to brood. They wage their battle to get their way stoically without silent resentment, fretting, moaning, or consternation. Brooding is an independent variable from absolutistic thinking and the agonistic tendency, but when each interacts with the other the combination causes far more problems, such as bitterness.

Brooding is comprised of cognitive, perceptual, emotional, and behavioral components. Cognitively, the brooder has imperative thinking (e.g., "This medicine must work.") that is reviewed over and over. When imperative thinking is not realized mental protests are waged against that unwanted circumstance ("Why? Why isn't this medicine helping?"). (Bear in mind, though, that the protest is not only due to the absolutistic thinking but also because of the agonistic nature of the individual, who will not let something drop and move on. Instead, that type of person continues to combat the source of displeasure.) The brooding replays the imperative thinking with a plaintive sadness, expatiating about what has gone wrong with life. Perceptual constancy adds to the problem by staying fixed on negative matter (e.g., rejection from others, loss of life's pleasure due to disease). The emotional component involves the dark, sullen, melancholy mood featuring sulking and self-pity that descends on the individual. Once the dismal mood envelops the individual, the brooder is more prone to think imperatively, that something must (or must not) occur. In essence, the relationship between brooding and thinking is reciprocal where each can influence the other. The behavioral component consists of sullen aloofness, withdrawal, or sluggish behavior. The agonistic tendency is then used to rally the brooder to overcome lethargy and battle on to get one's way. In this regard the brooder is at war with him/herself to persevere.

E. Castigation

The final variable to be considered provides an outlet for anger and hostility, in part created by the variables previously discussed. The anger is expressed as castigation against the object causing problems, or it is displaced onto other objects. The object can be the body that has failed to be cured or healed, God, life, health providers, or significant others.

It can take the form of blaming, hypercriticalness, and acts of meanness. The castigation seeks to punish, chastise, and inflict hurt, either in the person or within the patient's mind. The typical form of castigation is damning and berating, but it can also be done nonverbally through contemptuous sneers and disdainful looks, at other people or the patient's own ill, weakened, or dysfunctional body. The castigation can occur behaviorally as well, where someone is passive-aggressive or revengeful toward the source of pain (e.g., a patient overworks his body to punish it). In either case, castigation is hard to correct because it does feel good to gain revenge and punish.

Castigation is a cognitive-perceptual-emotional activity. Awfulizing conceives of the situation as the worst, which goes to fuel anger. Absolutistic thinking places demands on the situation to be different, and when that does not happen more anger is felt. Simultaneously perception stays fixed on the negative qualities and actions of the object that has caused the pain (e.g., the body, an employer). By maintaining that narrow, negative focus on the enemy or adversary, anger does not recede and in fact stays intense. Continuing to feel angry, the need for an outlet becomes paramount, which gives vent to castigation. Once in place as a tendency, it only causes the person to feel worse about him/herself or other people, which incites the tendency to brood.

CCT deals with castigation as a maladaptive coping strategy. It is a way to handle anger by giving it a voice and outlet. In this regard it siphons-off frustration. However, its means of doing so (e.g., revenge-seeking, severe criticism) keeps the person immersed in resentment. It causes counter-reactions in others that in turn ignites a desire for further revenge.

In summary, each of the variables in the irrational, maladaptive coping skill (IMCS) interact with one another. *If the agonistic nature, the tendency to brood, and the urge to castigate are not present, then health providers will have a much easier time resolving the presenting problem in a much shorter amount of time.* There will be much less bitterness if any at all.

To make this point, two case examples will be presented. Each is a hemodialysis patient suffering from chronic renal failure. Each has been taking dialysis for several years, several times a week, for several hours a day. In addition, there are other demands placed on each patient, such as good skin care, and dietary and liquid restrictions. Each patient is most tired of his demanding regimen, feels overwhelmed by it, and wants it to end somehow, someway.

Case Study: Ben

Ben is frustrated by all the time that dialysis takes. He is bitter about his life and depressed. He is easily disappointed by any act of the staff or other patients that cause him problems, or by any delay in getting him connected to a dialysis machine. He has a "problem exclusion" belief and engages in absolutistic thinking and awfulizing: "I should not have gotten kidney disease. I should not have to incur this lifestyle of spending my days in such a boring way. My life is awful and it should be better than it is. It should not have taken the turn that it has taken." Ben then evaluates his situation as a calamity and rates it as awful. Viewing his life that way he then feels severely depressed.

His therapist uses cognitive restructuring to treat his irrational thinking. The therapist first identifies Ben's response to his disease—bitterness about renal failure and not finding a kidney donor. Ben's problem exclusion thinking is then identified and the full implications of it are elucidated: "Ben, what I hear you say is, 'I should not have gotten sick. I should only be healthy and only have healthy kidneys. That is how my life was supposed to go. I was not meant to be ill. Other people can get ill but not me. I should be treated differently by life or God.' " Hearing this, Ben concedes that his thinking does not make sense.

To help him change his thinking, objective countering is also employed to help Ben make a philosophical switch. Ben is a very emotional person, so the therapist counters that tendency with a cool, non-emotional, logical argument. He reasons with Ben, "You may want to be special, but is anyone granted an exclusion from life's misfortunes?" The intent is to increase Ben's objectivity and stop demandingness about how life should have gone for him. Logic is able to persuade Ben to switch his philosophy to accept the fact that "bad things do happen to good people." Ben is able to see that he has had a maladaptive personal philosophy that contributes to his distress.

To treat Ben's irrational evaluation that his situation is awful, the therapist teaches him relativistic thinking. Ben's situation is placed on a continuum from extreme awfulness to mildly undesirable. He discusses with Ben other situations that could have befallen him and Ben evaluates those situations, using the above continuum. This gives him an objective perspective on his situation. Ben does concede that he only has a "mildly awful" to "fairly undesirable" situation that could have been worse, given the many complications that arise from chronic renal failure.

Another technique is used to show the central role of thinking in causing bitterness. To further facilitate a change, the therapist gives Ben a ritual. The therapist writes down Ben's irrational thinking and has him say it on odd days of the week whenever he becomes agitated about being ill and being in dialysis. That shows Ben how his thinking leads to a more intense negative response. On even days of the week Ben recites a self-instruction dialogue that includes a rational self-talk about kidney disease. Ben is told to chart how he feels at the end of each day after reciting each dialogue. After two weeks he admits that his irrational thinking causes more pain.

Treatment is prolonged, though, due to Ben's tendency to slip into brooding when he does not get what he most wants. This appears to be a biologically caused problem and not just a consequence of his absolutistic thinking. He has been a brooder since childhood. While intellectually he concedes that his thinking is irrational he nevertheless drifts back into it at times because of what Sharoff (2002) calls "positional slippage." To treat this problem, the therapist has Ben use rational-emotive imagery (Maultsby, 1984; Wessler & Wessler, 1980), where he sees himself not feeling upset and feeling calm while receiving dialysis. He then identifies thoughts that helped him have a less negative feeling. That allows him to form a self-dialogue to be said while receiving dialysis treatment: "It is unfortunate that this has happened to me. I don't like it one bit, but it is not the worst thing that could have happened to me. It's not really terrible because terrible would be dying and I am able to live with the aid of dialysis." Over time this way of thinking is able to decrease the amount of time Ben spends brooding.

Because Ben is not an agonistic individual, he does not push to fight against his misfortune. CR is able to help him drop his imperative thinking that life should have treated him differently. Overall, his awfulizing, absolutistic thinking, and brooding were the main factors that needed to be addressed. Once they were changed, he was willing to abandon his irrational coping strategy of disallowing his disease.

Case Study: David

Now, let's compare Ben to David, a fellow dialysis patient. Like Ben, David evaluates his situation as awful and has similar absolutistic thoughts. Like Ben, David is depressed about how he spends his days hooked up to the dialysis machines, laments that life has not been fair to him, and feels angry, resentful, and disillusioned about how his life has gone for him. He too actively disallows his disease and protests against it vociferously.

Initially the therapist uses the same cognitive restructuring tactics with David as he did with Ben. The therapist brings out David's special person thinking. David concedes that his thinking is irrational but that does not change his tendency to condemn his body and Life for causing his illness (Life is capitalized because David relates to it as a person who has meant to personally harm him). David stays steadfast in disallowing his disease. "I hear what you say that I am stuck in protest about getting sick. You are right. I lead one hell of a life and I do fight against living this way. I won't accept this damn disease."

The therapist works to inculcate relativistic thinking, that David's situation is bad and unfortunate but not terrible. David steadfastly disagrees. The therapist tries to make David realize that other ways of thinking could make him feel better. The therapist uses the method of difference technique (McMullin, 1986), telling David, "There are people in dialysis who are not nearly as miserable as you are. What are they saying to themselves that allow them to be that way?" Along with that the therapist employs solutions-oriented therapy (de Shazer, 1985, 1988). He asks David when he does feel happier and David is able to find times when that occurs.

However, he has no real inclination toward working to install others' helpful mind-set or the one he has when he does feel better, saying instead, "Feeling better about my dismal situation is not my goal." David remains disgruntled about his lot in life. He cannot shake his anger about his bondage to the dialysis machine that he hates but needs in order to stay alive. He angrily responds to the therapist's tactics, "You don't get it. You want me to feel better about having this disease and adjust to it. I won't. I want out of this mess I am in. Period. I hate being a dialysis patient. I don't want my life. Get it?" While David often thinks of suicide he maintains that he will not take that step so he is doomed to stay miserable as long as he has kidney disease.

The therapist tries a different tactic. He uses responsibility-taking. He asks David to take responsibility for causing himself to feel depressed by thinking irrationally. David readily does this. He admits that he knows that he makes himself feel worse but does not care. David, like many difficult, rigid, stubborn patients, has understanding of his problem but emotionally stays stuck in his depression, while admitting that his thinking is faulty. He admits that it is not written that he will receive fair treatment in life, but he still is angry that he has not gotten it. Overall, David makes little progress in treatment, largely due to his agonistic nature along with his tendency to brood and castigate. He cannot stop himself from mentally condemning Life and those not afflicted with disease. He is in combat with Life and God for shortchanging him, and excoriates them for giving him such a horrible existence. He remains bitter and frustrated with little hope for his future.

The therapist now switches tactics. He realizes that trying to convert David into becoming a rational thinker will rob him of his coping strategy of being agonistic toward Life, damning it, and protesting his situation. While his agonistic nature is maladaptive and causes him extensive unhappiness, it is his way of coping. He uses self-pity to comfort himself and his complaining does give him an outlet for his anger. He feels momentarily better after berating God, health providers, and significant others.

The therapist now moves to directly treat David's maladaptive coping strategy, the main reason for his resistance to change. The therapist uses two therapeutic strategies from CCT to address his resistance. Each strategy employs paradox and focuses on the patient's chosen coping response.

The first strategy works to help David become more adept in using his maladaptive coping strategy. He is trained to be **a "better" agonistic individual**. *In practicality, David is encouraged to stay disgruntled and miserable but to do it more proficiently.*

Step one involves highlighting how *David disallows his disease, by hating and condemning it. The intent is to vividly increase David's awareness of how he operates, to learn how he pursues his coping strategy hour by hour. He has David phenomenologically describe how he feels as he goes through his day. He wants David to be keenly aware of what it is like to be an agonistic, brooding individual, to know what he gains and loses by being that way.*

In step two, the therapist prescribes David's agonistic coping strategy. "You seem to get something out of it and you have no other way of managing your emotions." Specifically, the therapist encourages David to become better at protesting and combating against Life. The therapist identifies David's executive beliefs that direct his coping strategy of disallowing disease. They are:

- *Focus on daily losses from having the disease.*
- *Discredit and lambaste Life as part of the protest against disease.*
- *Stay sad to show Life that it has done a foul, rotten deed to me.*
- *Focus on others' shortcomings and problematic behavior to notice how their behavior causes me trouble.*

The therapist then directs David to practice these executive beliefs actively but stay miserable as he does it, to show Life how it has harmed him. Similar to Milan family therapy, his thinking is revealed and then he is told not to change (Boscolo et al., 1987).

However, the therapist adds to this strategy by employing a paradoxical coping skills orientation. The therapist questions David's ability to stay miserable. "Staying miserable when things go wrong is not a really good test of your ability to stay dejected. Anyone can be miserable when their life goes wrong. If you really want to show Life and God how horrible they have made your life, then you will need to become miserable even in enjoyable, pleasant situations. That will really show Life what it has done to you." David is then asked to participate in **"misery training,"** *where he will* endure *a series of pleasant activities but derive no satisfaction from any of them. He is asked to seek out situations that most people find pleasurable (something he does not presently do) but purposely not enjoy himself while in them.*

Thus, David is prescribed his maladaptive coping strategy. This is a compliance-based paradoxical strategy (Seltzer, 1986), where change is facilitated by complying with a prescription demanding that he continue doing irrational, dysfunctional behavior. By doing so he may realize the folly of pursing his maladaptive coping strategy ("Look at what I have done to myself!"). The strategy also places David in a double-bind. If he complies he exposes himself to pleasurable situations that may make him feel better. If he defies the strategy and does not stay miserable but oppositely enjoys himself he also benefits.

The therapist then teaches David how to stay miserable. A self-instruction dialogue is developed to ruin his fun. The dialogue contains the statements David already uses to stay miserable. A prescription is given to focus on negatives in the situation (e.g., noticing poor service in a very good restaurant) instead of positives (e.g., the great food in the restaurant). He is asked to engage in catastrophic thinking (which he already does regularly), by imagining worst-case scenarios for his Life. Whenever David notices that he feels any pleasure, he is asked to deliberately scale down his degree of pleasure using the above tactics. A monitoring system is installed to have David rate how successful he was at staying dejected.

In addition, a restraining strategy (Seltzer, 1986; Weeks & L'Abate, 1982) is employed, whereby David is restrained from making too much progress because that would challenge his agonistic nature. "You may find yourself at times feeling happy but that is not good. You need to hold back because you may not be ready to give up your anger toward Life right now." When David complains about his existence, the therapist encourages him to feel his pain even more, to make that stronger case to Life about how rotten it is for causing him to be deprived. After several weeks of encouraging David to stay miserable, David returns not complaining as much and feeling happier. He is choosing to defy the paradoxical prescription.

The therapist then suggests an alternative strategy to David to continue the war against Life. The therapist suggests living well as the best revenge. That will show Life that it has not hurt him and that he has risen above it in the end. David is not sure that he wants to switch to this pursuit. To treat his ambivalence, the therapist recommends a ritual from Milan family therapy (Boscolo et al., 1987). On odd days of the week David is told to practice misery training, and on even days of the week David is supposed to practice living well to gain revenge against Life. On those even days, he is to enjoy Life to the fullest.

To enjoy Life, he is taught the coping skill of **savoring** *(Sharoff, 2002). He shows David how to enjoy moments to the fullest as part of his revenge against Life, by increasing his awareness of each positive moment. A new combative strategy is devised, where David feeds himself self-instructions to encourage happiness, which coincidentally circumvents the desire to brood. The strategy of enjoying life also addresses his tendency to castigate. If he should focus on the faults of his wife and friends for being "bad" to him, to demonstrate to Life that he is living well, he must overlook their faults and not be upset about their behavior.*

In summary, by recommending that David become a better agonistic medical patient, he drops many of his maladaptive, non-utilitarian ways of thinking and acting. He adjusts to the life of a chronic illness patient. When that happens his therapist is able to utilize a straight-forward coping skills model in which he is taught skills openly, such as **assimilation of suffering**, **frustration tolerance**, *and* **disappointment accommodation**.

This case is presented to demonstrate the need to be eclectic and switch cognitive-behavioral tactics when necessary. David has a solution for his problem of being a dialysis patient, which includes absolutistic thinking, awfulizing, an agonistic strategy of combating with Life, brooding, and castigation. The problem is that his solution has become his problem. In that case, a second order change is necessary, to use the terminology of Watzlawick et al. (1974), that addresses his maladaptive "solution." A coping skills approach to paradoxical treatment is utilized and over time that overcomes his resistance to change.

How would traditional cognitive restructuring work with David? It would recommend more of the same—what Watzlawick et al. (1974) term a first order change approach: keep disputing, keep countering the patient's irrational thinking, but do it more vigorously (Ellis, 1993). CCT recommends that when that approach produces little change, then cognitive restructurists should instead switch to a skills orientation that may include a paradoxical tactic.

SUMMARY

Bitterness is one of the dominant feelings experienced by medical patients. Cognitive restructuring would deal with it by seeking to change absolutistic thinking and the tendency to awfulize. CCT would treat bitterness by focusing on a particular combination of skills that together cause pathology. That combination is termed an irrational, maladaptive coping skill. It is composed of a tendency for extreme evaluative ratings, insistence, an agonistic tendency, brooding, and castigation. Patients who have this response become more problematic in treatment. They frequently need a paradoxical form of treatment. A case example of one such patient, David, is provided.

References

Bandura, A. (1969). *Principles of behavior modification.* New York: Holt, Rinehart, and Winston.

Bandura, A. (1977). Self-efficacy: Toward a unifying theory of behavioral change. *Psychological Review, 84,* 191–215.

Bandura, A. (1997). *Self-efficacy: The exercise of control.* New York: Freeman.

Beck, A. (1963). Thinking and depression: 2, theory and therapy. *Archives of General Psychiatry, 10,* 561–571.

Beck, A. (1976). *Cognitive therapy and the emotional disorders.* New York: International Universities Press.

Beck, A., & Emery, G. (1985). *Anxiety disorders and phobics: A cognitive perspective.* New York: Basic Books.

Beck, A., Freeman, A., & Associates (1990). *Cognitive therapy of personality disorders.* New York: Guilford Press.

Beck, A., Rush, A., Shaw, B., & Emery, G. (1979). *Cognitive therapy of depression.* New York: Guilford Press.

Benson, H. (1975). *The relaxation response.* New York: William Morrow.

Benson, H., Beary, J., & Carol, M. (1974). The relaxation response. *Psychiatry, 37,* 37–46.

Berg, I., & Miller, S. (1992). *Working with the problem drinker.* New York: Norton and Co.

Berg, I., & Gallagher, D. (1991). Solution focused brief therapy with adolescent substance abusers. In T. Todd & M. Selekman (Eds.), *Family therapy approaches with adolescent substance abusers* (pp. 93–111). Needham Heights, MA: Allyn and Bacon.

Boscolo, L., Cecchin, G., Hoffman, L., & Penn, P. (1987). *Milan systemic family therapy.* New York: Basic books.

Burns, D. (1980). *Feeling good: The new mood therapy.* New York: Signet Book.

de Shazer, S. (1985). *Keys to solution in brief therapy.* New York: Norton.

de Shazer, S. (1988). *Clues: Investigating solutions in brief therapy.* New York: Norton.

de Shazer, S. (1991). *Putting difference to work.* New York: W. W. Norton.

Dobson, K. (1988). *Handbook of cognitive-behavioral therapies.* New York: Guilford Press.

Dobson, K. (2001). *Handbook of cognitive behavioral therapies* (2nd ed.). New York: Guilford Press.

Dobson, K., & Block, L. (1988). Historical and philosophical bases of the cognitive behavioral therapies. In K. Dobson (Ed.), *Handbook of cognitive-behavioral therapies* (pp. 3–39). New York: Guilford Press.

Dryden, W., & Ellis, A. (1988). In K. Dobson (Ed.), *Handbook of cognitive-behavioral therapies* (pp. 214–273). New York: Guilford Press.

Dryden, W., & Ellis, A. (2001). In K. Dobson (Ed.), *Handbook of cognitive-behavioral therapies second edition* (pp. 295–349). New York: Guilford Press.

D'Zurilla, T., & Goldfried, M. (1971). Problem solving and behavior modification. *Journal of Abnormal Psychology, 78,* 107–126.

Edwards, W. (1954). The theory of decision-making. *Psychological Bulletin, 51,* 380–417.

Ellis, A. (1962). *Reason and emotion in psychotherapy.* Secaucus, NJ: Lyle Stuart.

Ellis, A. (1971). *Growth through reason.* North Hollywood, CA: Wilshire Books.

Ellis, A. (1985). *Overcoming resistance.* New York: Springer.

Ellis, A. (1993). Vigorous RET disputing. In M. Bernard & J. Wolfe (Eds.), *The RET resource book for practitioners* (pp. II, 7). New York: Institute for Rational-Emotive Therapy.

Ellis, A., & Abrams, M. (1994). *How to cope with a fatal illness.* New York: Barricade Books.

Ellis, A., & Bernard, M. (Eds.). (1985). *Clinical applications of rational-emotive therapy.* New York: Plenum Press.

Ellis, A., & Grieger, R. (Eds.). (1977). *Handbook of rational-emotive therapy.* New York: Springer.

Ellis, A., & Harper, R. (1975). *A new guide to rational living.* North Hollywood, CA: Wilshire Books.

Ellis, A., & MacLaren, C. (1998). *Rational emotive behavioral therapy.* San Luis Obispo, CA: Impact Publishing.

Fennell, P. (2001). *Chronic illness workbook.* Oakland: New Harbinger Publications.

Fisher, R. (1991). *Getting to Yes: Negotiating agreement without giving in* (2nd ed.). New York: Viking Press.

Fordyce, W. (1976). *Behavioral methods for chronic pain and illness.* St Louis: Mosby.

Fordyce, W., & Steger, J. (1979). Chronic pain. In O. Pomerleau & J. Brody (Eds.), *Behavioral medicine: Theory and practice.* Baltimore: Williams and Wilkins.

Goldfried, M. (1980). Psychotherapy as coping skills training. In M. Mahoney (Ed.), *Psychotherapy process: Current issues and future directions* (pp. 89–121). New York: Plenum.

Gordon, D. (1978). *Therapeutic metaphors.* Phoenix: Meta Pub.

Gordon, D., & Meyers-Anderson, M. (1981). Phoenix: Meta Pub.

Guidano, V. (1988). A systems, process-oriented approach to cognitive therapy. In K. Dobson (Ed.), *Handbook of cognitive-behavioral therapies* (pp. 307–357). New York: Guilford Press.

Holmes, D. (1984). Meditation and somatic arousal reduction: A review of the experimental evidence. *American Psychologist, 39,* 1–10.

Hycner, R. (1985). Dialogical Gestalt therapy: An initial proposal. *Gestalt Journal,* Vol. VIII, 23–49.

Jacobson, E. (1938). *Progressive relaxation* 2nd ed. Chicago: Chicago Press.

Jacobson, E. (1972). *You must relax* (4th ed.). New York: McGraw-Hill.

Kanfer, F. (1970). Self-regulation: Research issues and speculations. In C. Neuringer & L. Michael (Eds.), *Behavior modification in clinical psychology.* New York: Appleton-Century-Crofts.

Kelly, G. (1991). The psychology of personal constructs (Vols. 1–2). New York: Routledge. (Original work published 1955).

King, M., Novik, L., & Citrenbaum, C. (1983). *Irresistible communication.* Philadelphia: Saunders.

Lang, P. (1977). Imagery in therapy: An information processing analysis of fear. *Behavior Therapy, 8,* 862–886.

Mahoney, M. (1988). The cognitive sciences and psychotherapy: Patterns in a developing relationship. In K. Dobson (Ed.), *Handbook of cognitive-behavioral therapies* (pp. 357–387). New York: Guilford Press.

Mahoney, M. (1995). The continuing evolution of the cognitive sciences and psychotherapies. In R. Neimeyer & M. Mahoney (Eds.), *Constructivism in psychotherapy* (pp. 39–65). Washington, DC: American Psychological Association.

Mahoney, M., & Arnkoff, D. (1978). Cognition and self-control therapies. In S. Garfield & A. Bergin (Eds.), *Handbook of psychotherapy and behavior change* (pp. 689–723). New York: Wiley.

Mahoney, M. Thoreson. (1974). *Self-control: Power to the person.* Monterey, CA: Brooks/Cole.

Marlatt, G. (1985). Relapse prevention: Theoretical rationale and overview of the model. In G. Marlatt & J. Gordon, *Relapse prevention* (pp. 3–71). New York: Guilford Press.

Martin, T., & Doko, K. (2000). *Men don't cry . . . women do: Transcending gender stereotypes of grief.* New York: Brunner/Routledge.

May, R. (1950). *Meaning of anxiety.* New York: Ronald Press.

Maultsby, M. (1984). *Rational behavior therapy.* Englewood Cliffs, NJ: Prentice-Hall.

McMullin, K. (1986). *Handbook of cognitive therapy techniques.* New York: Norton and Co.

Meichenbaum, D. (1977). *Cognitive-behavior modification: An integrated approach.* New York: Plenum.

Meichenbaum, D. (1985). *Stress inoculation training.* New York: Pergamon Press.

Meichenbaum, D., & Jaremko, M. (1983). *Stress reduction and prevention.* New York: Plenum.

Melzack, R., & Wall, P. Pain mechanisms: A new theory. *Science,* 1965, 50, 971–979.

Miller, S., & Berg, I. (1995). *The miracle method.* New York: W. W. Norton.

Neimeyer, R. (1985). Personal constructs in clinical practice. In P. Kendall (Ed.), *Advances in cognitive-behavioral research and therapy* (Vol. 2). New York: Academic Press.

O'Hanlon. W. (1987). *Taproots.* New York: Norton.

O'Hanlan, W., & Weiner-Davis, M. (1989). *In search of solutions: A new direction in psychotherapy.* New York: Norton.

Pelletier, K. (1977). *Mind as healer, mind as slayer.* New York: Dell Publishing.

Perls, F. (1972). *In and out the garbage pail.* New York: Bantom Books.

Perls, F., Hefferline, R., & Goodman, P. (1951). *Gestalt therapy.* New York: Julian Press.

Poppen, R. (1988). *Behavioral relaxation training and assessment.* New York: Pergamon Press.

Polster, E., & Polster, M. (1973). *Gestalt therapy integrated.* New York: Vintage Books.

Rehm, L., & Rokke, P. (1988). Self-management therapies. In K. Dobson (Ed.), *Handbook of cognitive-behavioral therapies* (pp. 136–166). New York: Guilford Press.

Rokke, P., & Rehm, L. (2001). Self-management therapies. In K. Dobson (Ed.), *Handbook of cognitive-behavioral therapies second edition.* New York: Guilford.

Rosch, E. (1973) Natural categories. *Cognitive Psychology, 4,* 328–350.

Rosch, E. (1975). Cognitive representations of semantic categories. *Journal of Experimental Psychology: General, 104,* 192–233.

Rosch, E., & Mervis, C. (1975). Family resemblances: Studies in the international structure of categories. *Cognitive Psychology, 7,* 573–605.

Rosch, E., Mervis, C., Gray, W., Johnson, D., & Boyes-Braem, P. (1976). Basic objects in natural categories. *Cognitive Psychology, 8,* 382–439.

Salkovskis, P. (1996). *Frontiers of cognitive therapy.* New York: Guilford.

Schultz, J., & Luthe, W. (1969). *Autogenic training (vol.1).* New York: Grune and Stratton.

Selekman, M. (1999). *Pathways to change: Brief therapy solutions with difficult adolescents.* New York: Guilford Press.

Seltzer, L. (1986). *Paradoxical strategies in psychotherapy.* New York: Wiley and Sons.

Selye, H. (1976). *Stress of Life.* New York: McGraw-Hill.

Sharoff, K. (2002). *Cognitive coping therapy.* New York: Brunner/Routledge.

Sharoff, K. (2004). *Coping skills for managing chronic and terminal illness.* New York: Springer.

Sheikh, A. (1983). *Imagery: Current theory, research, and application.* New York: Wiley and Sons.

Snyder, C., Cheavens, J., & Michael, S. (1999). Hoping. In C. Snyder (Ed.), *Coping: The psychology of what works* (pp. 205–231). New York: Oxford University Press.

Snyder, C., & Dinoff, B. (1999). Coping: Where have you been? In C. Snyder, *Coping: The psychology of what works* (pp. 3–20). New York: Oxford University Press.

Spivack, G., Platt, J., & Shure, M. (1976). *The problem-solving approach to adjustment.* San Francisco: Jossey-Bass.

Tomm, K., & White, M. (1987, October). *Externalizing problems and internalizing directional choices.* Paper presented at the Annual American Association for Marriage and Family Therapy Conference, Chicago, IL.

Watts, A. (1965). *The way of Zen.* New York: Random House.

Watzlawick, P., Weakland, J., & Fisch, R. (1974). *Change.* New York: Norton.

Weeks, G., & L'Abate, L. (1982). *Paradoxical psychotherapy: Theory and practice with individuals, couples, and families.* New York: Brunner/Mazel.

Wessler, R., & Wessler, R. (1980). *The principles and practice of rational-emotive therapy.* San Francisco: Jossey-Bass.

White, M., & Epston, D. (1990). *Narrative means to therapeutic ends.* New York: W. W. Norton.

Wine, J. (1981). From defect to competence models. In J. Wine & M. Smye (Eds.), *Social competence* (pp. 3–36). New York: Guilford Press.

Wolpe, J. (1958). *Psychotherapy by reciprocal inhibition.* Stanford, CA: Stanford University Press.

Wolpe, J. (1969). *The practice of behavior therapy.* Oxford: Pergamon.

Wolpe, J. (1973). *The practice of behavior therapy,* 2nd ed. New York: Pergamon Press.

Zeig, J. (Ed.) (1980). *A teaching seminar with Milton H. Erickson.* New York: Brunner/Mazel.

Zinker, J. (1977). *Creative process in Gestalt therapy.* New York: Brunner/Mazel.